Advance

"Highly recommended...a loving, much needed story of hope."

Liane Gentry Skye
> *Author, Turn Around, Bright Eyes,*
> *Snapshots from a Voyage Out of*
> *Autism's Silence*

"...straight from the heart!"

Mary Ganguli, MD
> *Professor of Psychiatry,*
> *University of Pittsburgh*

"...a memoir of extraordinary power...
resonates deeply"

Robert A. Naseef, PhD
> *Psychologist and author of Special*
> *Children, Challenged Parents*

"A touching story about parents' love..."

Cheryl Carmin, PhD
> *Professor of Psychiatry*
> *University of Illinois–Chicago*

"Inspirational and moving..."

Eva Ritvo, MD
> *Chair, Department of Psychiatry,*
> *Mount Sinai Medical Center,*
> *Miami Beach, Florida*

For the Love of Rachel

For the Love of Rachel

A Father's Story

David Loewenstein, PhD

Enalan Communications, Inc.
Fort Lauderdale, Florida

For the Love of Rachel

Published by:
Enalan Communications, Inc.
804 SE 14th Street
Fort Lauderdale FL 33316

www. enalan.com

+1-866-357-9920
+1-954-337-1860

ISBN 10: 0-9791943-4-2
ISBN 13: 978-0-9791943-4-2
LCCN: 2007926922

Manufactured in the USA.

Contents

Foreword

"Premature labor," "borderline viable," "fetal compromise"—no young couple anticipates ever having to hear these words. Yet prematurity is on the rise in the U.S. With increasing frequency, couples hear these words from obstetricians and neonatologists, a breed of pediatrician whose existence most of them have never heard of until those frightening moments when it becomes clear that a pregnancy is in trouble.

One such couple, Susan and David Loewenstein, and I, a neonatologist, connected in a special way with the birth of their daughter Rachel. Being a part of the medical team that helped care for Rachel in the first year of her life allowed me to do what I know best: to help tiny and fragile infants survive. In return, the friendship that developed between her parents and me allowed me the privilege of learning up close about what happens after a premature baby, once thought too small to survive, leaves the hospital. I learned what is asked from the child, the parents, the extended family, and the community. Rachel's story, as lovingly told by her father, takes us into the experience of one set of parents who overcame many obstacles to become what so many take for granted, a family.

Rachel's story is humbling, because all the medical heroics performed in the first year of her life become inconsequential when compared to the courage and fortitude she has shown in dealing with challenges every day.

I applaud her parents for wanting to share her story, and hope it will serve as an inspiration to others facing the same choices. For those of us who care for these tiny infants and their families on a daily basis, knowing what awaits them after discharge can only make us more caring and compassionate.

Shahnaz Duara, MD
Miami
April, 2007

Acknowledgments

Many people came together to make this book a reality. First, I want to thank my beloved wife Susan and my precious daughters Rachel and Amy. Their lives have been a true inspiration for anyone fortunate enough to know them. My parents Arline and Jack Loewenstein have always been there for me as role models of love, integrity and compassion. My dad has spent his whole life overcoming and prevailing against adversity, and I can't think of Rachel's tremendous strength without also thinking of the grace and dignity with which my father faces life's obstacles. My friend the late Dr. Andy Guterman continues to be a great inspiration to me.

Family is an essential part of our lives, and grandparents Doris Berkell, Gerald and Mildred Berkell and Arline and Jack Loewenstein have always helped and supported us when we needed them. Aunt Fran and Uncle Kevin Rafferty, Aunt Linda and Uncle Gabriele Brega and Cousins Jennifer, Michael, Kyle, Daniel and Alex have also loved and supported us every step of the way.

I am particularly grateful to the University of Miami/Jackson Memorial Hospital NICU. Drs. Shahnaz Duara, Emmalee Bandstra, Maria Buch, Magaly Diaz-Barbosa, Maritza Torres, Donald Buckner and Lisa Plano and scores of other physicians, nurses and healthcare professionals were a part of our extended family for nine months and have our gratitude.

My fellow faculty members in the Department of Psychiatry and Behavioral Sciences at the Miller School of Medicine at the University of Miami and my colleagues at the Wien Center for Alzheimer's Disease, particularly Dr. Ranjan Duara, at Mount Sinai Medical Center, Miami Beach, Florida helped our family through a most difficult time and have supported the creation of this book from its beginning.

Writing this book would not have come to fruition without the encouragement, wisdom and guidance of Dr. Ray Ownby, my excellent editor and publisher at Enalan Communications, and Tony Guzman's editorial assistance. My thanks also go to my friends and colleagues Drs. Eva Ritvo, Elizabeth Crocco, Amarilis Acevedo and Mary Ganguli for their helpful suggestions and comments on earlier versions of the manuscript.

Susan and I also very much appreciate the help of the Dan Marino Center in Weston, Florida, United Cerebral Palsy of South Florida, Dr. Sandy Rizzo, Educational Consultant, and Ms. Brenda Butler. The teachers and students at Coconut Palm Elementary School have been wonderful. We also thank all of the other friends, speech and occupational therapists, teachers and other individuals who have cared for Rachel and so many other children with special needs. To our friends who traveled with us to China to bring Amy home, we will never forget you!

Finally, we are grateful for the many parents and families of developmentally challenged children whom Susan and I have gotten to know over the years. These individuals as well as those who strive to improve the health and the quality of life of our children are true unsung heroes who deserve both our respect and admiration.

Chapter One

BORN TOO SOON

CERTAIN MOMENTS IN LIFE are indelibly etched in our memory. They may involve great joy or sorrow or a unique mixture of many different emotions. No matter what their nature, our lives are transformed and we are never the same. For me, the most profound moments of my life happened on the first day of November in 1995. It was just past 11 o'clock at night and I found myself led by a young nurse through a maze of winding hospital corridors. Eventually, we came to a set of large white double doors. The nurse quietly pushed one of the doors open and motioned for me to enter the room. I moved a few steps forward and took a deep breath. What I saw before me was to change my life and the lives of all of my family forever.

Lying in a tiny incubator, bathed by a bright light, I saw my newborn daughter Rachel. She weighed just 18 ounces and would have fit into the palm of my hand. White gauze covered her tiny unopened eyes. Her skin was so thin and translucent that it seemed as if I could see the bones and underdeveloped organs that lay underneath. Rachel's arms and legs were jerking spasmodically and it seemed as though she were writhing in pain. She was surrounded by countless machines with wires, tubing and needles attached to her tiny body.

I noticed the barely palpable whooshing sound of the ventilator that filled one of her lungs with oxygen. Rachel's other lung had collapsed after birth and she was fighting an infection that had ravaged her entire body. She was barely clinging to life. I studied her severely underdeveloped features. To a casual observer she probably would have appeared more like a horribly disfigured baby monkey than a human being. However, I knew that this precious life belonged to the daughter my wife and I had so very much wanted.

Stunned with anguish and disbelief, I saw the doctors and nurses running back and forth to attend to our child. It was difficult to keep my composure as the tears filled my eyes. I struggled to remain clear headed and focused since it was essential that I do everything possible to help our baby. A doctor and a nurse brought over papers to be signed to give permission for the necessary treatment. Whatever the risks, the medical professionals would do whatever they could to help save our daughter. I learned that Rachel would be vigorously treated with an antibiotic therapy. I spoke to the lead doctor, a neonatologist specializing in high-risk infants. He was quite concerned that not enough oxygen was being delivered to my daughter's blood. In addition, he was worried about the functioning of Rachel's underdeveloped organs. It was, he said, simply too early to know if she would survive. After learning this, and watching Rachel for a time, I knew that I had to get back to my wife. Susan had just gone through the ordeal of her life and needed my strength and support.

A normal human pregnancy usually requires 38 to 40 weeks, or about nine months. It takes that much time for a child to be sufficiently nurtured in the womb to fully develop her brain, lungs and other vital organs. At just 23 weeks gestational age, four months early, Rachel simply had run out of time. Her lungs weren't ready to function and her eyes weren't ready to see. She was simply a work in progress that had been abruptly stopped after being little over half completed.

Rachel had been in the womb for just 20 weeks when Susan noticed a watery leakage that she feared was amniotic fluid. She was rushed to the hospital where a weakness in her cervix was discovered. It could not bear the weight of the growing fetus. The amniotic sac was protruding into the birth canal and Susan was about to have a miscarriage. The doctors rushed Susan into surgery where they desperately tried to push the sac back into the womb and to place a stitch to help prevent our daughter's birth. During the following weeks, Susan battled heroically to maintain her pregnancy. Unfortunately, infection took hold of both mother and daughter and, three weeks later, Rachel was brought into the world by cesarean section.

At the time Rachel was born in November of 1995, almost no babies had ever survived after fewer than 23 weeks gestation. Given her prematurity and the extent of her complications, we had been told by the OB/GYN before her delivery that Rachel had less than a 5% chance of survival. As a fetus, Rachel had been protected and nurtured in Susan's womb. Now she lay squirming under a heat lamp, surrounded by a mesh of wires connected to the machines that were keeping her alive. I could not help but focus on the uncontrollable torturous and flailing movements of her tiny limbs. Rachel seemed to grimace in agony under the bright bilirubin light. Periodically, her mouth would open slowly as if she desperately wanted to scream but couldn't. What had once been the quiet and tranquil serenity of her mother's womb had now been replaced by the sound of the ventilator and the beeps and buzzers of the other machines that continuously monitored Rachel's vital signs.

I found it difficult to leave my daughter, but I also felt compelled to get back to Susan. She had been sedated and was burning up with a fever caused by the same infection that threatened Rachel. I found her lying under a white sheet on a gurney in the recovery room. Her face was pale and sweat beaded her forehead. I took her hand and squeezed it as she slowly opened her eyes. I was transfixed. Even on the worst day of her life, Susan was beautiful. She squeezed my hand feebly and anxiously asked, "How is she?" She held her breath as she waited for my answer. I tried to remain composed.

"The doctors are doing everything that they can for her," I replied. "We just have to pray." I paused for a moment, and then went on. "I think that you should see her."

Susan struggled to find her words. "I just can't see her like this." As a loving husband and clinical psychologist, I instinctively knew that Susan should see our daughter. If Rachel were not to survive, Susan would never forgive herself if she had not seen her baby while she had the chance. My wife also seemed to know that she had to see her child in spite of her fear. She needed to bond with the tiny being that had been inside her and to see the daughter that she had fought so hard to bring into this world.

A very kind nurse had overheard us and went to get a Polaroid camera. She would take a picture of Rachel and help prepare Susan for what she was about to see. It was one of the most difficult things anyone could ask a new mother to do.

After seeing the picture, Susan began to have second thoughts about whether she could go through with seeing our baby. I looked into her frightened eyes and told her that I was afraid that she might have regrets if Rachel were not to survive. We both intuitively knew how important it was for Susan to see our child in order to achieve closure in case the worst were to happen.

Susan took a deep breath and softly said to the nurse, "I need to see her...please." Susan's voice trailed off as she softly squeezed my hand. The nurse adjusted the gurney so that Susan was more comfortable and began to wheel her toward the room with Rachel's incubator. I leaned down and gently kissed my wife's forehead. As we entered the room, my heart ached as I heard the wails of grief as my darling wife of three years set eyes upon her newborn daughter for the first time.

Susan stared helplessly as the child that she had tried so hard to conceive and keep in her body squirmed under the bright light in her incubator. Susan wanted so much to touch Rachel and to hold her. She would have given her life to fiercely protect her daughter, but here she lay on a gurney powerless to protect and to comfort the infant who only a few hours before had been safely inside her womb. After several minutes, the experience of watching her struggling child became overwhelming for Susan and we left. Susan looked at her daughter, perhaps for the last time. She was a young mother fighting the exhaustion of childbirth and the debilitating infection that flowed through her body. The medications were kicking in and my wife drifted in and out of consciousness.

I went with Susan to the hospital room that had just been assigned to her. She seemed to be burning up with fever. I asked the nurse to get my wife some water and I wiped the sweat from her forehead.

"I am glad that I saw her," Susan began. "I love her so much." Her eyes welled up with tears and I held her until, exhausted and drained, she drifted off to sleep. I then went to check on Rachel. Little had changed. I signed more papers consenting to still more procedures. The attending physician told me once again that Rachel's situation was extremely critical and that it was "touch and go." I just sat with my daughter and watched her, feeling more helpless than I had ever felt in my entire life.

By the time I returned to Susan's room about an hour later, she had awakened and looked terrified. "David," she gasped, "When

I saw that you were gone and you didn't come back, I thought something had happened to Rachel and you couldn't bear to tell me." I took her head into my arms and stroked her hair as I let her know that nothing had changed. We held each other for the longest time, both agonizing silently over whether our infant daughter would survive through the night.

Chapter Two

THE BEGINNING

I NEVER BELIEVED that I could ever meet someone as wonderful and special as Susan. As a boy of twelve or so growing up in southern Florida, I made extra money mowing lawns for our neighbors. During these jobs I would ponder my future. I often wondered what my future wife might be doing at a particular moment. Many a sprinkler was run over as I daydreamed about my future.

My parents had a strong and happy marriage and considered themselves to be best friends and soul mates. It was exciting to think that somewhere in the world was someone I would meet and with whom I would eventually fall in love. I wondered what her name might be and about her interests. Was she a blonde, brunette or redhead? Did she live in Miami or even in Florida? I was a shy, gangly and awkward preadolescent. It was hard for me just to talk to girls, much less ask one to go out on a date. I wondered if my future wife were dating someone. Whoever it was, I absolutely hated him.

Even then, I knew that when I grew up I wanted to be in a profession where I could communicate with and help people. Sometimes I imagined being an attorney, arguing in court on behalf of a client who had been wronged. Perhaps I would become a psychologist like my mother, devoting my life to helping people wrestle with challenges that stood in the way of their happiness and fulfillment. Whatever my future occupation, I knew that I wanted to be married with perhaps two or three children. I did not know at the time that it was much easier to find a suitable career than a suitable wife.

After finishing college, I was accepted to graduate school in psychology and I completed my doctoral degree at Florida State University. To finish my training as a clinical psychologist, I went on to an internship at the

University of Washington School of Medicine in Seattle.

I was fortunate in that upon completing my internship someone brought my name to the attention of the Chair of the Department of Psychiatry and Behavioral Sciences at the University of Miami School of Medicine. At 26 years of age, and a newly minted Ph.D., I became one of the youngest faculty members in the department. I was thrilled to be working in the hometown where I had been born and raised. Over the next several years, I developed a cognitive assessment laboratory devoted to Alzheimer's disease and over time became the Director of Psychological Services and Neuropsychological Laboratories at the Wien Center for Alzheimer's Disease and Memory Disorders at Mount Sinai Medical Center on Miami Beach. My career was in high gear, and it seemed I was ready to achieve all the things I wanted to.

I did not meet my wife, though, until after my 32nd birthday. By then I had been promoted to the rank of Associate Professor and I was trying to get funding for my laboratory from the National Institutes of Health. There was little time to eat or sleep, much less date. Some of my friends were convinced that I would never find a life partner. My life was consumed by my drive for achievement and by my perfectionism. Not only did I maintain a perfectionist attitude towards my work, but I wanted my future life partner also to be perfect. She had to be beautiful, intelligent, genuine, compassionate and interesting.

Of course, the incongruity here was that somehow this ideal person would have to be attracted to and fall for me. I was, after all, a quite ordinary looking fellow who was a driven workaholic. My many years of academic training had not left much time to cultivate pursuits that might be interesting to others. Few people were interested in spending large amounts of time pondering the inner workings of the human brain, talking about the development of test measures that were sensitive to early cognitive decline in patients with memory problems or the newest statistical techniques available for the analysis of data. I remained on the academic fast track and my social life simply took a back seat.

The manner in which Susan and I first met was due in large part to our mothers. My mother had met Susan's mother at a family gathering through a cousin with an impressive record for matchmaking. She duly noted that each of our mothers had a child who was single and then let them brag about their "remarkable children." At the time, I was dating an elementary school teacher, certainly nothing serious, but then again, I did not have much time for anything too serious.

One evening, the telephone rang as I was poring over some computer printouts of data analyses from a recent study.

"David," my Mom began, "I just met the loveliest woman who has a daughter that just got out of a relationship."

I cut her off. "Mom, I'm already dating one person, and I've gone out a few times with other people. I'm not really interested in meeting someone else."

My mother persisted. "But she sounds like a wonderful girl, and she's waiting for your call."

"Mom," I protested, "I didn't ask for you to promise her mother that I would call."

Mom was not buying this at all. "David, be a gentleman! This poor young lady is expecting your call and she'll be terribly disappointed if you don't at least try to contact her."

I knew I had lost this argument. In addition to being a keen child psychologist, my mom knew me like a well-read book. The guilt about hurting this person's feelings would make me pick up the telephone and make that call. Being shy myself, I knew how awful it felt to anticipate a telephone call that never came. Still, I could not help feeling somewhat hesitant. My well-meaning parents had occasionally tried to arrange dates for me in the past and, unfortunately, their batting average was not too good. I promised Mom that I would call and continued what was otherwise a very pleasant conversation. I never expected anything to come from my call to Susan other than an awkward attempt at conversation and an exchange of social pleasantries.

In reality, Susan was hardly holding her breath for a telephone conversation with me. She was a busy registered nurse who had recently left an unfortunate relationship and was grateful to finally have some time for herself. Conducting home visits for the elderly involved a considerable amount of driving and she had a busy case load. While her mother wanted her to begin dating again, Susan was not particularly enthusiastic about the idea. She was just settling down in a new apartment overlooking the waters of Biscayne Bay with her recently acquired kitten Patches. Why should she concern herself with dating when she was thoroughly enjoying her newfound freedom and the serenity of her surroundings?

I was unusually nervous as I dialed the number my mother had given to me. The phone rang several times, with no answer. Finally, an answering machine picked up and I was relieved to be able to leave a message with a brief introduction and my telephone number. At least I could say that I had done my duty. This young lady would know that I had made the effort to call and now the ball was in her court. Perhaps she would call back in several days as dating etiquette dictated, or maybe she would not return my call at all. Having met my obligation, I returned to the array of fascinating data spread out before me.

Twenty minutes later the phone rang. Fully immersed in my work, at first I did not notice it ringing in the other room. By the fourth ring, it was too late. My machine began picking up a message.

"Hi, this is Susan. Sorry that I didn't get your message, but I was taking out the trash."

"Hello," I stammered, picking up the receiver. "How are you?"

The next hour passed wonderfully and effortlessly. Instead of the awkwardness I usually felt in this kind of encounter, I soon felt as if I had known Susan for years. She seemed genuine, spontaneous and very sweet.

I normally would have asked her out for lunch or perhaps a drink after work but there was something quite unusual about her. She sounded so nice and decent that I felt that no matter what I wanted to at least have dinner and get to know her. We made a date.

The night of our date rolled around and I struggled to try to find Susan's apartment complex. Unlike some men, I will be the first to admit that I am not particularly good with directions. That night was certainly no exception. It was ten minutes after 7:00 PM, the time I was supposed to meet Susan in front of her complex, and I was still trying to find her building. Fortunately, I finally found an understanding security guard in a parking garage who gave me directions.

I was now over 20 minutes late. "Good first impression," I muttered to myself. Thoughts of guilt began swirling in my head as I visualized Susan being extremely upset waiting for me to arrive. Maybe she would think that I had stood her up.

Several cars were ahead of me waiting to pick up people standing on the curb in front of Susan's building. As I pulled up, I could not help but notice a beautiful brunette in a white dress with long beautiful legs. Again I muttered to myself, "I'm sure *her* date will pick her up on time."

As people in the cars ahead of me continued to pick up their passengers, this particular beautiful young lady continued to wait by the curb. She was the only person left waiting when my car pulled up. I hesitantly rolled down the window and asked meekly, "Susan?" She flashed a shy smile and I instantly knew how people felt when they hit the lottery. The woman with the warm, wonderful personality that I had spoken to on the telephone was simply beautiful.

I took Susan out to my favorite Italian restaurant and after dinner we went for frozen yogurt. I could not believe that I felt so comfortable and relaxed with this gorgeous creature. Most scientists and researchers spend their days relying on facts and data. They simply do not believe in fate or in magic. This night, however, was magical and I was smitten. Unfortunately, it took a while longer for Susan to feel the same way about me. Thanks to the encouragement of her sister Fran, Susan did not let me scare her off. Within two months we were engaged and within seven months we married.

I had spent years in graduate school learning that human beings often go through an infatuation phase in the early stages of a budding relationship during which they project their hopes and illusions onto another person. Many of these projections involve previous or unresolved relationships with other people in their lives, including their parents. Of course, the danger of such illusions is that, as time goes by, each person begins to experience the other as they really are rather than as they had imagined. All of us are merely flesh and blood and cannot possibly live up to or meet others' idealized standards, needs or expectations. Part of the continued growth and maturity of a relationship is learning to love and to accept another person for who they are rather than blaming them for not having attributes that had only been our own projections. As long as people relate to an idealized or projected image rather than an actual human being, it is impossible to both accept and appreciate another's unique individuality.

Many of my friends who were psychotherapists warned me about how quickly Susan and I were moving in our relationship. "Take it slow, David. If this is meant to be, it will develop over time." At this age and point in my life, however, I knew what I wanted. Deep down and despite my commitment to my profession, I really wanted to settle down and have a family just as I had imagined when I was 12 years old and mowing lawns. I remember a conversation I had with my Dad at that time. He somehow did not think I was quite as crazy as everyone else did. You only had to see the expression on his face when my mother entered the room to know that he and I had something very much in common.

As time went on, each hour that I spent with Susan made me fall more head over heels for her. She was loving and accepting in ways that I had never imagined. When I was nervous, I would become self-conscious and tended to ramble, but it never seemed to bother her. I was extremely disorganized and misplaced things, but Susan remained unfazed. Talking to her was as effortless as breathing. Her humor and spontaneity were simply exhilarating. During our second date, I remember driving Susan home and dreading that awkward moment when it was time for the parting kiss. I hesitantly asked if I could kiss her. Her playful response was "on the cheek or on the lips?"

Susan had previously been married. In spite of having been hurt in the past, she had not lost her spirit and did not relinquish her idealism. She was down to earth and natural. Beneath her effervescence was a deep sensitivity and compassion. Like a diamond, Susan had many facets that sparkled. She shined brighter every hour that I was with her.

Susan and I had gotten pretty tipsy on our third date. I was six feet tall and she was five feet three inches. I mistakenly thought that I could drink her under the table, but I had not accounted for differences in our individual metabolism of alcohol. After only a few drinks, my nose was completely numb. I was thankful to be in the company of a nonjudgmental RN. As the night wore on, we snuggled together before a small bonfire on the outside deck of the restaurant bar and talked about our love for children.

That night I told her about my best friend Andy, a neurologist and psychiatrist in my department who had taken me under his wing when I had joined the faculty of the medical school at just 26. He was barely 40 when he succumbed to a brain tumor that took him away from his wife and small children.

I had not gotten over his death and recalled his haunting words as he called me at work late at night and said, "Dave, hasn't my illness taught you anything? Go home and start to enjoy life." He continued, "Find a woman of substance who will be a good mother to your children." I told Susan all about Andy; how he had been one of the most personable members of our faculty. Andy had said that I was a graduate of his "dare to be wonderful course."

As his illness progressed, it was increasingly more difficult for many people to see and spend time with him. Nonetheless, his family and closest friends remained. I talked about the devotion of his wonderful wife and how after late nights at work they would feed me dinner and let me sleep on their couch. As I talked, Susan stared at me with her big, beautiful brown eyes. We talked of our childhoods, our hopes and our fears. That night we agreed that if we had a daughter, we would name her Rachel. Her middle name would start with an A for Andy—that was Susan's idea. Our daughter's name would be Rachel Andrea.

Chapter Three

THE JOURNEY BEGINS

After Rachel's birth, while we waited in the hospital room, I gently kissed Susan's forehead. She was burning with fever. I tried my best to reassure her as I held her small hand in mine. Susan was totally exhausted and gradually drifted off to sleep. I thought back over the path that had led us to this moment.

For the last two years we had been desperately trying to have children. When we were unable to conceive, we had consulted with specialists who had sent us to more specialists. We discovered that Susan had problems with an irregular menstrual cycle and blockage of her fallopian tubes. Moreover, my sperm count was well below normal and the experts opined that Susan could never become pregnant through natural means.

The tension and gloom on the faces of the men and women sitting and waiting for their fertility consultations was often heartbreaking. For their entire lives, these people had just assumed, as we had, that they were never going to have any difficulties having children. Everyone in the waiting room was now dependent on advances in medical technology to help them to fulfill their dreams of becoming parents. The despair in the waiting areas of these specialists' offices was sometimes so thick that it seemed that you could cut it with a knife. In each fertility clinic that we visited, there were beautiful fish tanks and relaxing scenes pictured on the walls. These diversions however, did not hide the palpable anxiety and sometimes despair that permeated the room.

Susan and I felt particularly sorry for the women who were alone. In speaking with these women, we were frequently told stories of multiple in vitro fertilization cycles where the husband's only involvement was to make a donation. During our many visits to doctors, Susan and I continued to notice how few men there were relative to women. It seemed unjust that much of the burden of these procedures was borne by the woman who wanted to fulfill her dream of becoming a mother. As we spoke to our fellow patients in the waiting room, it was amazing how important it was for them to have a biological connection to a new life. We were inspired by the courage and dedication exhibited by these people to fulfill their dream of bringing children into the world.

After visiting with many specialists, taking hormone shots and other fertility medications became a natural routine for Susan. She taught me how to administer injections by practicing on oranges that we had in the refrigerator. Over time, we came to realize that the only realistic chance for us to have children was to consider a procedure whereby single sperm cells would be injected into individual eggs and then embryos would be grown in a petri dish. We went to Virginia and underwent the first round of in vitro fertilization. Unfortunately, on that first cycle, Susan became over-stimulated on the hormones. As a result, the embryos that had been produced needed to be frozen for later implantation. A number of these embryos, consisting of only several cells, were not viable when Susan and I returned four months later to have them implanted. Despite our heartfelt prayers and the hormone injections, none of the embryos that were implanted attached to Susan's intrauterine wall. The procedure was grueling both physically and psychologically. Susan and I briefly looked into adoption but were not selected from among several applicants by a birth mother that was going to have a baby. After this disappointment, we decided that we would try one last round of in vitro fertilization near our home while looking into other potential avenues of adoption.

In what would be our second and last in vitro fertilization attempt, Susan had four of our largest, most mature embryos introduced into her womb. A couple of weeks later, we received the wonderful news that one of the embryos had successfully implanted and that

Susan was at last pregnant. We could barely contain our excitement about finally becoming parents. Our family and friends, who had been so supportive during these cycles of in vitro fertilization, were now ecstatic. We would read books about child development and each day I would dutifully give Susan a progesterone shot to reduce the possibility of miscarriage. We felt that we had so much love to give to a child and we simply could not imagine life any other way.

The pregnancy progressed with excitement as well as morning sickness. An amniocentesis revealed that we were going to have a healthy baby girl. I could not imagine two parents who could be happier. We began to plan setting up a nursery and to buy baby clothes. Each of our sisters was looking forward to planning a wonderful baby shower. After such a rocky beginning, things finally seemed to be falling into place.

During her 20th week of pregnancy, Susan went to the bathroom and experienced what her training as a nurse suggested might be the leakage of amniotic fluid. I drove her to the obstetrician and the tests confirmed that her assessment had indeed been correct. Rushed by ambulance to the hospital, a skilled obstetrician worked feverishly to stop the miscarriage and to push back the amniotic sac that had begun to protrude from Susan's cervix.

We would later learn that Susan had a condition referred to as "incompetent cervix," meaning that it could not bear the weight of the growing baby. Many times this condition is diagnosed only after a miscarriage has occurred. However, we were fortunate and the obstetrician managed to push the amniotic sac high enough to close Susan's cervix with a stitch called a cerclage. Although the amniotic sac was forced back into Susan's body, the leakage was caused by what the obstetrician found was an irreparable tear. The only hope to avert miscarriage was complete bed rest and fetal monitoring in a hospital with all of the most modern equipment.

Susan's physician sat down and explained to us that the primary goal was to try to keep the baby inside of her for another 7 to 12 weeks. Although she would be born quite small, a baby at 27 to 32 weeks had much better odds of survival. Unfortunately, because of the tear in the amniotic sac, there were two major problems. First, a certain level of amniotic fluid had to be present for the fetus to survive. At 20 weeks gestation, Rachel was not capable of surviving outside of the womb. Second, the tear in the amniotic sac left both our baby and her mother vulnerable to serious infection.

Susan was started on a vigorous regimen of antibiotic therapy and wore a device to monitor the baby's status at all times. She also endured uncomfortable bed positions and, at times, had to lie virtually upside down in order to relieve pressure on her cervix. Susan was still losing amniotic fluid and her family and friends, along with the wonderful hospital staff, helped her to get through each day.

By the end of the 22nd week of gestation, though, it was clear that Susan was not going to be able to carry the baby much longer and she was administered surfactant, a miraculous substance that had been developed with the support of the March of Dimes. Surfactant would allow our daughter's underdeveloped lungs to mature faster in case she had to take in air. Prior to the availability of surfactant, infants born at fewer than 25 weeks gestational age simply could not survive. On the morning of the exact day marking the 23rd week of gestation, Susan had an unusually uncomfortable pain in her abdomen and her monitor was showing increasing fetal distress. By nine o'clock that evening, Susan was eight centimeters dilated and was prepared for emergency surgery. The obstetrical surgeon on call found that Rachel was turned the wrong way and would have to be delivered by caesarean section. He sadly informed us that our daughter's chances of survival were minimal.

I held my wife's hand tightly as the incision was made into her abdomen, peering over the surgical curtain to see what was happening. I saw the surgeons cut away at the subcutaneous fat and then saw blood. The mood was somber as an increasing number of persons entered the operating room. Everything seemed to be going in slow motion and taking forever. Given the tenor of the conversation among the medical staff, we became increasingly worried that our daughter was lost. Suddenly, without warning, we heard a tiny, almost defiant cry. Every heart in the room was racing as a little bundle that Susan and I could not clearly see was passed to a neonatologist and hurried from the room.

I looked into Susan's eyes. There is perhaps no greater fear for a mother than harm coming to her child. As I held Susan's hand she implored, "Please David, check on Rachel, make sure she is okay." If only I had that power. Rachel was in extremely critical condition and the worst was yet to come.

Chapter Four

HOLDING ON
TO LIFE

THE FIRST COUPLE OF WEEKS of Rachel's life were touch and go. She had fallen to under a pound in weight, had a collapsed lung, and multiple infections were all taking their toll. We were constantly at Rachel's bedside as she received the first of many blood transfusions. Susan was able to pump breast milk into bottles to bring to the hospital. They had started to feed Rachel small amounts through a nasogastric tube. This was essential for getting her intestines to start to work properly. Her glucose levels were problematic and she had to be administered insulin. Rachel was still dependent on a ventilator because of her extremely underdeveloped lungs and if she lived, would remain on the ventilator for several more months. Her battles with infections were life threatening but it appeared that with the help of antibiotics Rachel had finally gained the upper hand. I kept a journal of her daily progress and by the 11th day of her life we finally had reason to be somewhat optimistic. In my journal I wrote:

November 12, 1995:

1) Blood transfusions have resulted in a platelet level of 90 up from 50;

2) Blood results show no sign of infection;

3) Weight 427 grams (0.944 pounds);

4) Lung stability has been up and down and chest x-ray shows scars and infiltration. Placed on steroids to reduce lung edema (swelling);

5) Doctors want to refrain from giving broad spectrum antibiotics because of risk of fungal growth;

6) Heart echocardiogram set for tomorrow to rule out PDA (patent ductus arteriosus, a common developmental abnormality of the heart in premature infants that may require surgery). Scheduled for a brain scan.

Rachel's eyes had been open for just two days. Susan thought that she had seen Rachel stick out her tongue. Every parent believes that their child is the most beautiful in the world and we were not exceptions.

By the third week of her life, with help from the antibiotics, Rachel had fought off a number of infections and seemed to be getting stronger. Nourishment was provided via a central line in her neck and she received medications through a needle attached to her right arm. During this time, our family kept a constant vigil by Rachel's bedside and offered us their love and support.

My friends and colleagues, Dr. Ranjan Duara and his wife Shahnaz, visited Rachel the first day that she was in the hospital. Ranjan was an accomplished behavioral neurologist specializing in Alzheimer's disease and we had worked together ever since I had joined the faculty at the University of Miami more than nine years before. Shahnaz was a neonatologist at the University of Miami School of Medicine/Jackson Memorial Hospital, or JMH. It was comforting to learn that some of Rachel's physicians had been Shahnaz's former residents and fellows and to know that our child was in the care of a highly trained group of professionals at a Level III neonatal intensive care unit (NICU).

Although Rachel's life hung in the balance during the first two weeks of her life, and despite the pessimistic evaluation of at least one of the neonatologists, our daughter held her own. Susan and I would visit Rachel in the hospital and gently touch her through the openings in the incubator. I would sing her songs hoping that somehow the love in my voice could comfort my daughter amidst the welter of flashing lights, the incessant beeps of the monitoring machines, and the needles and tubes inserted into her arms and neck.

It was inspiring to see the doctors, nurses and respiratory therapists going from incubator to incubator trying desperately to help these tiny and fragile babies hold on to life. There was little room for error and a poor decision could easily prove fatal. With all of the evils that existed in the world, it was wonderful to see how many people were committed to finding good in preserving and enhancing life. The medical professionals raced back and forth not to secure money, power or prestige, but from a simple desire to help the tiniest of God's creatures who were battling for their lives.

It was the night before Thanksgiving and the telephone rang at our home. On the other end of the line was one of Rachel's neonatologists.

"There's been a complication," he began hesitantly. "We think that Rachel has had a thrombosis or a spasm of the artery in her right arm—the one that was connected to the needle carrying IV fluids. Our vascular surgeons are examining her now but her entire arm is beginning to turn black."

"What are our options?" I asked, my head starting to spin.

"Well, we can try to treat her with TPA [a blood thinner], but it is highly unusual to use it with a child this young and we run the risk of bleeding into the brain. We have never treated an infant this sick with TPA and we would have to do it in consultation with one of the specialists at Jackson Memorial Hospital."

I asked him why she could not be transported to JMH, since they were the experts in this kind of treatment. The neonatologist replied that Rachel's condition was too critical to move her. I quickly called one of those specialists whom I knew personally. Drs. Shahnaz and Ranjan Duara were about to catch a cab to go to the airport. Thankfully, Shahnaz picked up her cell phone when I called. I quickly explained the situation.

"David, we have experience with TPA. You need to get Rachel to JMH. I will talk with her doctor and make the arrangements," Shahnaz told me. She continued, "You and Susan should meet the ambulance at the hospital."

Shahnaz addressed the other doctor's concerns about transporting Rachel to JMH. The ambulance hurried from Fort Lauderdale through the streets of Miami with a neonatologist and a nurse attending to Rachel. She had already received an initial dose of TPA when she was rushed into the NICU of JMH where we were met by the Chief of Service.

Rachel's right hand to her forearm was black and the entire arm to her shoulder was a mixture of purple and gray. The Chief shook his head sadly and said that he would do everything that he could to save the arm. Rachel was bundled up and placed into a tiny incubator. There were rows and rows of incubators as far as the eye could see, each holding a precious human life. The technology was so awesome that it seemed as if we were in a science fiction movie. Sadly, this was not fiction; our daughter was in danger of losing her right arm.

The NICU staff and the TPA helped save Rachel's right arm and hand but she lost her second finger and part of her thumb. Several other blackened fingers on her right hand withered away and eventually fell off. Her hand was covered in gauze and constantly treated to help avoid infection. On November 26th Rachel weighed 405 grams or slightly less than 14.3 ounces—about nine-tenths of a pound. In addition to the TPA, she was also urinating constantly because of the Lasix (a diuretic, or water pill) that was administered along with her blood transfusions.

Over the next several days, Rachel began looking quite sluggish and she had difficulties associated with a high triglyceride count and insufficient oxygen in her blood. She also had problems with regurgitation of food and her heartbeat would become slow (bradycardia) and irregular when she was handled. Rachel was started on a regimen of both antibiotics and antifungal medication, since she was suspected of having both types of infections. Over the next several weeks, she continued to battle the infections. One night we received a call from one of Rachel's physicians saying that she was afraid that the infection had gotten the better of Rachel.

For the next week, it was like being on a horrible roller coaster ride. At times it would seem as if Rachel were rallying and hours later she appeared to be fighting a losing battle. Susan would stay with Rachel during the day and then I would stay with her after work in the evenings. The outpouring of support from our close-knit family and friends helped us to get through, but, most of all, Susan's and my love for each other sustained us. Most relationships are not truly tested, at least not early on. However, with each new adversity Susan and I became more strongly united in our love for each other and for the love of Rachel.

Slowly, with treatment from our doctors and our support, Rachel's health improved. When she was at her sickest, her weight had dropped to a little more than 14 ounces. Now she was finally rebounding and her weight had increased to 24 ounces, approximately a pound and a half.

I visited her every day after work. After scrubbing in and donning a mask, I was able to hold my daughter and she seemed to like it when I sang to her. It may have been that when she smiled it was merely gas, but somehow I felt that I was able to connect with her. I participated in "kangaroo care," in which an infant is placed on the bare chest of his or her parent. The skin-to-skin contact seems to help the baby's heart rate and respiration. When I did it with Rachel, she looked calm and peaceful. At times I would look into her eyes, now open, and saw her soulful eyes staring back at me. I wondered what she made of all of this. How could she understand the constant intravenous tubes, the countless blood tests and the fact that she had to live in a tiny incubator?

We surrounded Rachel's incubator with pictures of the family, stuffed animals and toys that made soothing sounds similar to what she might have heard in the womb. Our mothers, fathers, brothers, sisters and friends all visited and lent their support. I got to know some of the other children and parents who were undergoing a similar ordeal and quickly came to realize that the illness of a child is a great leveler. Your race, religion, or politics did not matter. Whether you were rich or poor or whatever your station in life did not matter. A common experience and the love for our children brought us together. It was painful for us to see the parents, whom we met and had come to care for, experience setbacks. Some babies did not survive.

In spite of their hectic schedules and awesome responsibilities, the physicians, nurses, respiratory therapists, social workers and other healthcare professionals at the University of Miami/ Jackson Memorial hospital always maintained their humanity and respect for the children and their families. Everyone was on the same page: we were all there for our children.

Chapter Five

FROM BAD TO WORSE

A LITTLE OVER FIVE WEEKS had passed since Rachel was born and again, something was terribly wrong. Her belly was bloated and distended. Tests were ordered and our worst fears were confirmed. Rachel had necrotizing enterocolitus, a leading cause of death among premature infants. A top surgeon was called and agreed to operate.

When he opened her abdomen, he was distraught to find small holes throughout her small intestine. He considered patching the areas of dead tissue but too much damage had already occurred for this to work. It seemed hopeless.

Shahnaz, the NICU doctor, implored the surgeon, "I know this child and I know these parents. They are fighters. Keep cutting. Do anything that you have to do."

The surgeon continued to work against seemingly impossible odds. With the finest surgical skill he cut out one third of Rachel's small intestine, but in the end he could not remove or patch all the damaged tissue. After the surgery, the surgeon came to the small room where Susan and I were anxiously waiting.

He began slowly. "We did everything that we could but we just couldn't repair certain parts of Rachel's small intestine."

I needed something more concrete. "What is the probability that she'll survive?"

The surgeon shook his head and said, "I believe that it's clinically impossible." His voice trailed off. "Her chances of survival are perhaps one in ten thousand."

Susan and I were stunned. Thankfully, Shahnaz was there both to comfort and guide us. Rachel's condition continued to deteriorate and it appeared that she was in considerable pain. Shahnaz and the other physicians advised us that we could choose to help ease her pain by placing her in "comfort care." No life support would be removed but there would be no heroic efforts to keep her alive. If she faltered, we would let God take her.

Susan, I and the family held Rachel in our arms for possibly the last time. I sung her lullabies and tried to soothe her. Susan's mom, Doris, shook her head, saying that she just did not feel in her heart that Rachel was going to die. Susan's sister, Fran, put a gentle hand on her shoulder, saying, "Mom, we have to be realistic." Surrounded by the group of people who loved Rachel the most, we said our last good-byes.

Susan and I had rented a hotel room across from the hospital for those times we could not be away from Rachel or were simply too tired to make the 25-mile trip home. When we got to the room, we just held each other.

"I am so sorry, honey," I said softly to my wife. "She fought so hard."

Susan replied, softly weeping, "Oh God, I love her so much."

I thought about both Rachel's and our refusal to give up, but like so many things in life, much was beyond our control. I remember praying to God that whatever His will, I would accept it. I vowed that if Rachel were to survive, no matter what challenges lay ahead, we would love her unconditionally and use every resource at our disposal to support her and to help her reach her full potential. But if in God's wisdom, He wanted to take our daughter, I resigned myself to the fact that it was His will. Of course, God or the universe does not need anyone's permission to fulfill the destiny that awaits all living creatures. Hope and faith are things that we cling to in our darkest hours, desperately hoping that we are heard and understood amidst the din of all of the pain and anguish around us.

It had not seemed fair that Rachel had to spend her brief existence in so much pain, hooked up to machines, and stuck with so many needles that she looked like a pin cushion. However, neither was it fair that Andy was taken from his wife and children in the prime of his life, or that millions of people in the world live in poverty and squalor while others have more abundance than can ever be used in a lifetime. Acceptance is one of the most difficult aspects of living.

Susan and I tried our best to accept what lay ahead.

We returned to the NICU several hours later to find the doctors perplexed. Given Rachel's physical condition, it was expected that she would not have survived the night. A few hours later, our tiny daughter was still hanging on. The next morning the attending physicians were shocked to see Rachel still clinging to life. Shahnaz Duara ordered some blood samples to be drawn and later came back with an astonished look on her face. "This is not the blood of a dying baby."

Many of Dr. Duara's colleagues did not concur. Perhaps she was simply too close to this family and wasn't viewing things objectively. Shahnaz continued, "What if the baby's bloated belly is related to the positioning of the surgical drainage tube?" The doctors considered this possibility and monitored Rachel's condition throughout the day.

By that evening, Rachel was still fighting and Shahnaz's theory had gained some credence. The tube Shahnaz had mentioned was responsible for draining fluids that usually accumulate after surgery. It had been repositioned and Rachel's swollen belly looked a bit better. Somehow the holes in Rachel's small intestine that had leaked free air had sealed themselves over.

Within a week, Rachel's belly returned to almost to its normal size. The doctors and nurses who were veterans of the NICU were simply amazed. Rachel had been one of their sickest babies and had miraculously survived. Some people took to calling her "Miracle Rachel" or "Iron Rachel." Our baby was one tough cookie and was blessed with the strength to come back yet another time. I slowly rocked her in my arms as I sang our favorite song. Rachel's soulful eyes stared back at me and, for the first time, they looked content.

The next few months would prove to be an emotional roller coaster. At times Rachel would seem to be gaining ground. Then, she would have a setback, usually in the form of a life-threatening bacterial or fungal infection.

Many challenges remained. At the time Rachel had received surgery for the colitis, the doctors had performed an ileostomy in which her waste products were diverted to a small bag outside of her tiny body. She had to have more surgeries on her stomach because of adhesions (growth of scar tissue that can occur after surgery) and concerns about obstruction. Because of these difficulties, her small intestine could not be reconnected to her large intestine.

Rachel's brain scan showed that she had bleeding in the brain called an intraventricular hemorrhage. Fortunately, it was mild, and we prayed that there would not be significant brain damage.

On a routine eye examination it was discovered that Rachel had retinopathy of prematurity (ROP). This is a condition seen in about 16% of premature babies. ROP involves the abnormal growth of blood vessels in the retina of the eye. Left untreated, these vessels can cause retinal scarring, detachment of the retina and blindness. Specialists at UM-Jackson Memorial Hospital/ Bascom Palmer Eye Institute used laser surgery to correct the condition. She had a serious case of ROP and it was unclear how it would affect her vision. We were told that it was likely that Rachel would have some loss of vision and blind spots where damage had occurred.

Over the next several months, we came to know the nurses, other neonatologists and respiratory therapists who were so skilled and committed to the needs of the babies under their care. Each day Susan would come in for the daily weighing and we would take heart when Rachel would gain 10 or 20 grams. During Rachel's many bouts of infection in the hospital, we would despair as her weight dropped. It was a vicious cycle in which toxic bacteria would be treated with powerful combinations of antibiotics and then lower her good bacteria so much that she would develop major fungal infections. These then had to be treated. There were times when blood had to be taken every several hours and we wondered how many more places they could find on her tiny body to draw blood from and to insert the central line that would carry nutrition and medications into her system. Rachel had weighed barely 14 ounces when she was at her sickest, but gradually with IV supplementation she gained weight and became stronger.

The day that they moved our daughter from the area of the NICU that housed the sickest babies, Susan and I knew that she was finally out of the woods. Although Rachel would eventually spend a total of nine months in the NICU, the move to a step-down unit meant that we could now focus on the task of bringing our daughter home.

Chapter Six

REFLECTIONS

A s I sat by Rachel's bedside, I had many hours for reflection. Inside the hospital walls was a tremendous devotion to the preservation and enhancement of life. However, I could not but help think about the millions of children around the world who die each year because of poverty, malnutrition and lack of the basic immunizations that in the United States we take for granted.

Even in our own country, poverty, homelessness, lack of medical care and limited resources are devastating to many children and families. I wondered whether the world that my daughter was born into would be better than the one Susan and I had found. In a society consumed with winning, achievement and self-indulgence, I also wondered if the heroic babies in the NICU who survived this experience might be afflicted with physical and mental limitations. Would these children be embraced as the special and unique human beings they were, or be marginalized because they could not keep up with others? As terrible as their early lives had been up to this point, it was unclear whether this was just the beginning of the challenges facing them in a fast-paced society that seemed so intolerant of imperfection and weakness. What would become of the tiny creatures and their families in this room who had battled so valiantly for life?

The respect that everyone in the NICU bestowed on each infant and their families stood in stark contrast to many parts of the world where there is often disregard for the sanctity of life and the dignity of people. I looked in awe at the parents as they held their children and tried to encourage them, sometimes in languages and customs that were unknown to me. The differences between us were not nearly as important as our similarities. All of us were connected by the love and the bonds with our struggling children.

To build and to heal takes a much longer time than to destroy. It may take many years to build the smallest village, but it only requires a minute to drop a precision bomb on a community which will destroy it forever. Moreover, the money spent building that bomb could have been spent promoting life rather than rendering death and destruction. Constructing bridges takes considerably more effort than destroying them.

In a similar manner, turning one's back on the plight of others is often easier than rolling up one's sleeves and working for a common and workable solution. The many hours that I spent at Rachel's incubator caused me to reflect upon my own life and values. As I looked around the room, I was reminded of something I had read in the philosophy of Saint-Exupéry: *What is truly important is invisible to the eye.*

I remembered when my best friend Andy had been dying of a brain tumor five years before. He had not yet been 40 and had already accomplished a great deal in his young life. He had completed both psychiatry and neurology residencies and had also received a PhD in pharmacology. He had married a wonderful woman who was the love of his life and had two small children. He had a magnetic personality and people were drawn to him. I used to get calls from him late at night at work and he would tell me: "Stop living your life only to work. Get a wife and have a family."

I did not fully realize then what I now know—life is much more than meeting goals, attaining success, and being at the front of the pack. Life is about much more. It's about connecting with the people who are most meaningful to us, and it's about pursuing values that link us to others.

As I looked down on Rachel sleeping, I prayed that my daughter would have a chance for her life to unfold before her. I also recommitted myself to devoting more of my life to connecting with those things that are truly important: my wife and my daughter, my family, and the fellow human beings that I encountered on life's journey.

Rachel spent nine months of her early life in the NICU, the amount of time that most full-term babies spend in the womb. Because she had spent so much time in the incubator, I felt that it was very important for Rachel to be held. In retrospect, I don't know if holding Rachel was more for her or for me, but I suspect that it helped us both. During these many days and nights I developed a unique and special bond with my daughter. There was a spirit about her and a sparkle in her eyes that was awe-inspiring. She reminded me very much of my father, who was one of the strongest and most honorable men I have ever known

Rachel's grandfather, Jack Loewenstein, was sickly as a child and had suffered from bouts of rheumatic fever. To recover, he spent several years in bed at a time, the only treatment available at the time. His heart muscle was scarred, and he had once collapsed on the steps of his high school. Just a few months before the polio vaccine was discovered, he was diagnosed with this often fatal illness and many believed that he would not survive. His doctors later assured him that he would have to accept the fact that he would never walk again. Dad was unwilling to accept this fate and taught himself to walk, sometimes bursting blood vessels in his nose from the effort. Despite his battles with infirmity and a tumultuous home life, he married a wonderful woman, my mother Arline. She was more interested in the person underneath than the thin legs that were the result of polio. Dad worked his way up from being an engineer at a local television station to becoming a renowned acoustical engineer who developed one of the first underwater cameras of its kind.

He led a team of oceanographic scientists and spent a very productive career as a research scientist until he suffered a rare form of stroke caused by a spontaneous dissection of the internal carotid artery. In this kind of stroke, the inner lining of this critical blood vessel blocks the flow of blood to the brain. This combination of the stroke and post-polio syndrome left him in a wheelchair and he lost the use of his left arm. He remained, however, one of the strongest and most optimistic persons whom I have ever known. He was determined to keep his autonomy and continued to build telescopes, repair machinery and help blind and disabled persons to learn amateur radio.

To this day, Dad refuses to feel sorry for himself. Once when I asked him if he was bitter, he told me that he didn't have time for bitterness, saying, "Bitterness is the corrosive that consumes the container that holds it." In some of my darkest hours, my Dad would reach out to hug me and say, "Remember, David, life is like a game of golf. You may be on the green or in a sand trap. You have to play the ball where it lies."

Dad's attitude enabled him to succeed when it would have been easy to give up. His strength and positive attitude in the face of adversity taught me that it is not so much the obstacles that you encounter in life as how you respond to the challenges that you face. I knew that whatever Rachel faced in the days, months and years ahead, she would have to play the ball where it lay. I looked into her tiny face and saw the face of a warrior, like my father. I resolved that I would always be there for her, just as Dad had always been there for our family.

Chapter Seven

HOMECOMING

RACHEL RESPONDED to the supplemental nutrition supplied by the IV and grew bigger and stronger. At first she remained too small for regular baby clothes so Susan would buy clothes usually used to dress dolls from the local toy store. I may be a bit biased, but I think that Rachel was definitely among the most fashionable babies in the NICU. As the days passed, Susan would usually spend a large part of the day involved in Rachel's daily care. Since Susan was a skilled registered nurse, the nurses felt comfortable letting her participate in some of the minor aspects of her medical care. Rachel was blessed to have two primary nurses instead of one. I would come in later in the afternoons and the evenings to sit with my daughter.

Rachel eventually grew sufficiently large that she was given her own crib. It was exhilarating to see her reach for her rattle and stare in amazement at toys that had pleasant sounds and blinking lights. By her eighth month in the NICU, Rachel weighed more than five pounds. We were told that when she reached six or seven pounds, we would finally be able to take her home.

Susan and I happily prepared Rachel's room for her homecoming. In her early days, we had approached every weighing on the scale with dread because our daughter would often lose weight during her many life-threatening bouts with illness and infection. Now, however, these weighings were a source of excitement and joy. Every gram Rachel gained meant that she was that much closer to coming home.

Finally the day arrived when Rachel was to be discharged. She now weighed 6.2 pounds and was happily cooing and babbling in her crib. She seemed to sense the excitement surrounding her impending discharge. The morning lab results on that day, unfortunately, showed an abnormality and we had to wait an agonizing two additional days before Rachel could leave the hospital at last.

Finally the day came when Susan and the nurse placed Rachel in a bassinet and dressed her in her finest clothes. Rachel was a little overwhelmed by the excitement and stared at her injured right hand, something that she did whenever she became stressed or bored. I went to retrieve the car from the parking garage. I pulled up to the curb, we loaded our precious cargo into the car, and made the 25-mile trip north to Rachel's new home.

One of the most challenging aspects of Rachel's care after her homecoming was insuring that the ostomy bag that contained her waste products was kept continually clean and secure. We were not as skilled as Rachel's nurses in placing the bag over the stoma that protruded from her belly. Susan and I also had to wake up every two hours in the middle of the night to feed her Progestimil, an unpleasant smelling predigested formula. Rachel slept in our room in a portable crib next to Susan to facilitate these regular feedings, and so that we could constantly monitor her activity. Rachel seemed to enjoy her new surroundings and thrived. Within ten days, she had grown an amazing 11 ounces! Fearful of infection, we allowed family members and friends to visit Rachel only one person at a time. Our daughter seemed to enjoy the attention and amenities of her new home.

For the first several months after her homecoming, Susan and I experienced all of the joys associated with having a new child. Rachel loved being held and would coo and babble with delight as she would roll over in her crib and play with her many toys. I noticed that our daughter seemed to have a fascination with toys that were electronic and had lights and sounds. She did not have much use for stuffed animals. I had learned that her mother also did not seem to care for stuffed animals when we were dating. Not all things ran smoothly. Try as I might, I always had difficulties with replacing the ostomy bag after cleaning and was grateful that Susan was so proficient in meeting our daughter's medical needs. One thing I did well was burping my daughter after feeding, but then I had been well trained by her Mom.

In September of that year, Rachel began to have terrible difficulties with diarrhea and she suffered from dehydration. The doctors who had wanted to wait a year before reconnecting her intestine and bowels decided that it would have to be done immediately. Susan and I felt considerable posttraumatic stress as we had to readmit Rachel to the hospital for the surgery. It was especially painful to watch the medical personnel reinsert another central line. Fortunately, the surgery was a success and Rachel was able to return home for her first birthday.

Only our parents and immediate family attended Rachel's first birthday party. There was great joy in the festivities. She was surrounded by her parents, grandparents, uncles, aunts and cousins. One year after the terrible circumstances surrounding her birth, our daughter was finally home to stay.

The consensus of most experts is that temperament is inborn. Rachel had one of the sweetest temperaments that our family and friends had ever seen. Her disposition was continually sunny and she would smile readily. She loved playing with others and being held, but was equally content to play alone with toys in her crib. We had been somewhat worried that the many months of isolation in the incubator might cause Rachel to withdraw and have difficulties in relating to others. Nothing could have been further from the truth. Rachel enjoyed the presence of other people and loved interacting with those around her.

As time passed and Rachel grew, we learned that she had mild cerebral palsy. She did not walk independently until she was two and one-half years of age. The speech therapists who worked with Rachel were unsure whether she would ever be able to speak normally. Susan and I strongly believed in early intervention. This meant that Rachel was involved in all sorts of physical therapies, speech therapy (for chewing and swallowing problems), and occupational therapies (for learning to manipulate items with her hands). Because of problems in absorbing nutrients within her remaining small intestine, Rachel had regular appointments with her pediatrician and her gastrointestinal physician. Rachel was also monitored for her extremely poor eyesight and was prescribed glasses. She subsequently underwent eye surgery for strabismus, a condition in which weak muscles cause the eyes to cross.

At two and one-half years of age we took Rachel to a school that allowed her to receive even more therapies. The staff were entranced with Rachel's vibrant personality and infectious smile. For the next several years, she continued to receive her therapies at the school. It was a moving experience as Rachel graduated from school with the other special needs children. A number of her classmates were in wheelchairs and faced challenges that were even greater than those confronting our daughter. That evening was a celebration of all the hard work that the children had put into their rehabilitation, and to thank all of the parents, teachers and therapists who had supported them.

Susan and I had decided that we would send Rachel to the local public school. We were convinced that it was important to have as mainstream an education as possible as she entered kindergarten. Armed with the federal and state laws pertaining to exceptional student education and accompanied by my mom, who had been the supervisor for autistic programs for Dade County Public Schools, we attended a meeting with public school staff in which an individualized educational plan (IEP) was developed. Rachel entered a regular kindergarten class with an aide provided to support her educational needs. The new school had just been built in our area and had brought in a remarkable principal, Toni Weissberg. Ms. Weissberg took Rachel under her wing and assembled an outstanding team of special education consultants and teachers who worked with Rachel. Because of all of Rachel's special needs, no one knew for sure how this arrangement was going to work.

In the beginning, Rachel would become overwhelmed in the regular classroom. She would then become inattentive and act out. We had a number of meetings with the school's staff and it was their consensus that Rachel could only handle a few hours of kindergarten at a time. We wondered whether limiting her time in the class would be the best for Rachel and found a child psychologist to help out. She worked with the teachers and the school in developing behavioral programs and sticker charts and helped Rachel's wonderful aide.

As a result of everyone's effort and collaboration, Rachel became able to attend the entire day of kindergarten. We were also blessed that Susan's mom was a retired kindergarten teacher who could help out with projects. She had excellent suggestions and advice to enhance our daughter's learning. With everyone's help, Rachel kept up with kindergarten. The children in her class loved her and were very protective of her. If Rachel had a good day, everyone in the class would give her a round of applause.

The strong collaborative relationship between ourselves and the public school system helped to insure Rachel's success. It was Rachel herself, though, who touched something deep inside of all of us and made us determined that we would not fail.

Chapter Eight

A SPECIAL CHILD

UNDERSTANDING THE ISSUES of a special needs child is not only important to families affected by prematurity, genetic abnormality or developmental disability. The need to see each child as a unique individual is equally important for parents with developmentally normal children. Children have an array of temperaments and aptitudes, even when they come from the same family. The individuality of children dictates that the one-size-fits-all approach to child-care, child-rearing and education is not always desirable or appropriate.

It is often a challenge for parents of developmentally normal children to parent in accord with their child's unique constellation of strengths and weaknesses. The parents of children who were born too early, as well as those of children born full term but with genetic or physical abnormalities, confront a host of other issues as their child grows older. For example, physical limitations such as visual and hearing loss, as well as difficulties in ambulation, may make it difficult for children to access a full educational experience. Medical conditions and surgeries can also cause children to miss an excessive amount of school, making their academic work that much more difficult. We have all known of children with dyslexia, autism or attention deficit disorder who struggle to keep up with an educational curriculum. For children with these difficulties, coupled with an atypical physical appearance or physical limitations, academic problems may also be further compounded by limited social interactions that may interfere with their emotional growth and development.

Children with cerebral palsy, Down's syndrome, facial or limb abnormalities, severe visual or hearing loss or other conditions may be shunned by others because of their appearance. One has only to look at popular culture to appreciate our society's obsession with physical perfection. We hold high fashion models who are rail thin and have flawless skin as standards for beauty. The obsession with perfect ultrathin bodies has led to unhealthy eating habits and a growing epidemic of anorexia and bulimia. Many people spend hour upon hour in the gym sculpting their muscles to achieve an idealized image far beyond the amount of exercise needed for health benefits. Our society values and clings to youth through costly diet pills and other supplements, anti-aging creams, cosmetic surgery and other means which have become a multibillion dollar industry.

This striving for perfection and superiority is not merely limited to outer appearance but also affects our judgments of what it means to be a "successful human being." This can greatly influence how we think about ourselves and other people. Many people are driven to "keep up" with or to surpass "the Joneses" and live in larger houses, drive expensive cars, associate with people thought to have high status and send their children to the most prestigious schools. "Winning" has become the mantra of many people, constantly driven by their need for status and success.

Given these societal influences, the parents of a special needs child face a unique set of pressures. For Rachel, such apparently simple things as being able to chew food or put on clothing were major challenges. She went to numerous speech therapists who spent many hours teaching her to chew by trying food with different textures and performing simple exercises such as biting on a saltine cracker. Our daughter's inability to coordinate her chewing and swallowing was a serious concern since it placed her at a risk for choking and aspiration. Many times she would gag when food of a certain texture was simply placed on her tongue. If it were not for the many cans of formula which gave her vitamins and minerals, Rachel would have had to live with a tube in her stomach for feeding.

Her digestive problems associated with the "short gut" syndrome that resulted from her intestinal surgery led to challenges in toilet training. Difficulties with coordination and the loss of several digits on her right hand coupled with fine motor and visual problems often made it difficult for her to put on or take off clothing. These were just a few of the many challenges that were a part of Rachel's everyday life.

For millions of special needs children, simple acts of crawling, walking, dressing, speaking and bathing require as much practice and dedication to master as the training regimen of an Olympic athlete. When an amateur or professional athlete performs admirably on the playing field, he or she is often rewarded with a chorus of cheers. No fans cheer on, however, the special needs children engaged in their day-to-day struggles. Rather, there is only the quiet encouragement of supportive family, friends and therapists. The challenges that these children face are not known or appreciated by the average person. In fact, the effort required for them to do what many other children master easily is often immense and heroic. At stake is not a value on a scoreboard indicating whether a team has won or lost. The actual stakes are much higher. A special needs child's inability to master these fundamental skills can have a profound effect on their ultimate level of independence as well as their quality of life now and in the future.

For special needs children and their families, the arrival of each day presents a unique set of challenges. For some children the challenges are physical, while others struggle to communicate with words or have to spend their childhood learning to read or write simple words. Many parents legitimately fear that if their child cannot become independent they may have to be placed in an institution when the parents become older. Every loving parent dreams of launching a child who will be independent and make his or her own way in the world. Unfortunately, many parents of children with special needs are haunted by unpleasant images regarding their child's potential future. Equally worrisome for many families are the financial demands required to cope with an uncertain tomorrow.

The ability to accept the physical and

cognitive limitations of a special needs child requires that parents confront societal expectations regarding perfection and beauty. Those parents who are fortunate eventually come to understand that trapped beneath the child's physical and mental limitations lies a unique person who deserves love, nurturance and respect just as does any other human being. Whether born normally, imperfectly or too soon, each child is part of God's handiwork and a most worthy member of His universe. A person is no less human because of physical deformity or mental limitation. In fact, those who have special needs children or those who teach them often come to realize that the superficial evaluation of others based upon appearance and capabilities, such as how far someone can throw a baseball, fails to take into account each person's uniqueness. *What is truly important is invisible to the eye.*

We live in a complex, fast-paced society and have so many things competing for our attention that we often live our lives on "automatic pilot," never taking enough time to understand our underlying assumptions and core beliefs. We spend our lives relying on headlines or sound bites rather than understanding the complexity of a particular news story. All too often, it is easier to judge a book solely by its cover and we frequently judge style over true substance.

The parents of a child born prematurely or with a disability quickly come to understand that all of the assumptions that they had about normal development and their role as parents must be carefully re-examined. For a physically disabled child, developmental milestones such as walking and talking might be delayed for months and years. Sadly, they may not ever occur at all. Parents may look forward to introducing their children to new foods. This is not the case for a child who has difficulties chewing or is tube fed. Parents with healthy small children often share with other parents a camaraderie that develops into lifelong friendships. They share outings, play dates and get-togethers which are all rewarding aspects of the parenting experience. Because special needs children are different, other parents and children may feel unsure or uncomfortable in interacting with them.

Some parents of children without special needs experience discomfort in interacting with special needs children since they may serve as a reminder of just how vulnerable their own children could be to illness or injury. Unfortunately for the parents of physically and mentally challenged young children, the lack of companionship with other parents and friendship offered by other children often serves to increase their feelings of isolation. As a result, parents with special needs children frequently attempt to reach out to the parents of other special needs children.

It is these relationships that helped me to understand that in spite of the magnitude of Rachel's daily challenges, some families had to deal with far more than we could even imagine. It is truly amazing and inspiring to see these parents, sometimes single parents working full-time, driving their child to therapies and attending to their child's physical, cognitive and emotional needs. Our family faced many issues due to Rachel's difficulties in absorbing nutrients from food, her many visual and physical challenges, and her cognitive and emotional immaturity. Our burdens, though, were small compared to those of other persons whom we knew whose children were hooked to machines, nasogastric tubes, or who had profound developmental delays and mental retardation. If being a hero is defined as being selfless and fighting for a cause bigger than oneself, and courage is defined as doing what is honorable despite one's fears and trepidation, then these individuals are true heroes in every sense of the word. Silent and unrecognized, they are entrusted with the most important tasks in the world: caring for one of God's struggling children.

Susan's and my close relationship, the fact that I had a stable job and our family's steadfast support also made things somewhat easier. Many people that we knew with special needs children did not have these advantages. The stresses of having a child with developmental disabilities often tore away at the fabric of marriages, and a number of families did not have resources available to meet all of the costs associated with their child's medical needs. And then there were the parents who sat home alone, wondering what life would be like if their beloved child had survived.

Chapter Nine

A SISTER

T HE YEAR WAS 2000 and the new
millennium had just begun. Despite
the concerns of many regarding the potential effects of the change in centuries on our
computer-driven society, our civilization continued to function normally and we continued
with our daily lives. Four years had passed
since Rachel had left the NICU. Despite the
day-to-day challenges that came with her
special needs, Rachel remained delightfully
happy and content.

Susan and I came to accept that, given the
circumstances surrounding Rachel's birth, for
us having other biological children was out of
the question. We both loved children, however,
and wanted to have another child. Thinking
about this, our earlier insistence that we have
a biological child who had "sprung from our

loins" seemed unreasonable. Susan and I pondered what had driven us and so many people like us to go to such great lengths to conceive a child. More importantly, we thought that Rachel could benefit from having a sibling and, in turn, an adopted sibling could benefit from a loving family.

From the earliest days of humankind, there have been biological drives and social pressures to have children. This has an adaptive function, of course, since procreation is necessary for the survival of our species. Nature has aided in this process of procreation. Sexual attraction is pleasurable and ensures the renewal of the human race across the generations. Humans not only need to procreate but also need to protect the smallest creatures that they bring into the world. Biological and social factors help to explain why most people have such a positive reaction to a baby's face.

The social importance of having children also lies in the stigma historically accorded to women who were considered "barren" or "without child." This undoubtedly is connected to the pressures that women face in their roles as the bearers and primary caretakers of children. Even today, girls are more likely to be praised for playing with dolls than are boys, even though the boys will have the equally important task of being good fathers.

No one can deny that it is exciting for two people in love to think about having a child in their own image, a tiny being who will share their common genes, ancestry and characteristics. For many, maintaining the family lineage is a way to carry on beyond physical mortality. Privilege and fortune pass from one generation to the next because of no greater accomplishment than that an heir was born into the family.

In light of this historical perspective and the overt as well as more subtle societal pressures and social expectations, it is not surprising that many people experience a profound sense of despair and even shame when they have problems in conceiving a child. The burden is particularly hard on women, many of whom spent their entire lives believing that having a child was their destiny.

Susan and I had believed that having a child was the ultimate expression of our love. For us, parenting a child was one of our greatest responsibilities, as well as one of our greatest anticipated joys. Like so many other couples battling infertility, we had exhausted our emotional and financial resources in achieving our shared dream. Susan and I were fortunate in that the in vitro fertilization procedure was successful the second time around. By that time, though, we had decided that the toll that it took on Susan's body was simply not worth another attempt.

Our journey to several infertility clinics allowed us to meet many women who had undergone the in vitro fertilization procedure many times. They had spent years as virtual pin cushions receiving countless injections with many different types of hormones. They had spent hours undergoing these medical procedures to fulfill their dreams and those of their families. Despite their courage, some would never become pregnant and experience the joy of giving birth.

I vividly remember talking with one woman who had made more than ten in vitro fertilization attempts. She would receive treatment for four weeks or more at clinics far from her home, staying there alone while her husband attended to the family business. He would fly into town and donate his sperm and then she would pray that this would finally be the time when she would achieve her dream of becoming a mother. We heard too many of these stories during our attempts with in vitro fertilization. The tears and the pain involved simply made our hearts ache.

Our doctors had told us that Rachel's prematurity was unrelated to our problems with infertility. The cervical weakness experienced by Susan, we were told, is a problem experienced by many women who do not have problems becoming pregnant. Unfortunately, "incompetent cervix" is often diagnosed only after the loss of a pregnancy. A cervical stitch and strict bed rest had brought Rachel to the point where she had a chance for survival. We thought about the possibility of Susan becoming pregnant again, however, and decided that we had beaten the odds so many times that we might not be so fortunate in the future. Adoption became our only viable option.

At forty years of age, we were a little old for adoption through traditional routes. To be honest, we still had some sensitivity about not having been selected by the potential birth mother in our previous attempt at adoption. We had several opportunities to adopt special needs babies, but we felt that Rachel had so many needs that it would not be fair for her, the new baby or us to take on this added responsibility. As with Rachel, if one of our children were to be afflicted by illness or have special needs, Susan and I would go to the ends of the earth to provide for him or her. We had decided, though, that we would not take on another child with special needs.

In the back of my mind was another consideration. Susan deserved to know how it felt to have the more usual experiences, challenges and joys of motherhood. It was exciting to contemplate having a child who reached developmental milestones at the regular times, and to witness the more usual unfolding of a human being.

Susan and I were particularly touched by the situation in China where the one child rule has been instituted for some groups in many parts of the country. In China, boys provide a form of social security for their parents in their old age. When a woman marries, though, her obligation is to take care of her husband and his family. Parents who have a daughter and who are limited to one child face a very uncertain future for their old age. Over 100,000 Chinese girls are abandoned each year, mainly because of the one child rule and its implications. Since it is illegal to abandon a child in China, parents sometimes travel hundreds of miles to anonymously drop off a daughter at an orphanage, a fire station or some other place where someone will find her. The future of these little girls is often grim. Without family support, the best many of these little girls can hope for is institutional care and a menial factory job.

Our family and friends pointed out that since we came from European ancestry, perhaps we should consider Russian or Romanian adoption. Although the situation has changed, at that time Susan and I were both concerned about reports of the poor health of children from Eastern Europe. Moreover, at the time two separate visits were required to adopt a Russian child. Since Susan and I had decided that both of us would make any trip to visit an adoptive child and Rachel was not up to the rigors of travel, making two trips for a Russian adoption was out of the question. Over the next several months we intensely researched many different avenues of adoption but were undecided about what route we would eventually take.

It was July of 2000 when Susan excitedly came into the extra bedroom we use as an office, pointing to a page in the morning newspaper. In the paper was an advertisement stating that an organization that helped with Chinese adoptions would make a presentation in the South Florida area for prospective parents. We decided that this was an excellent way to obtain further information on adoption and we made plans to go to the meeting. Grandma Doris stayed with Rachel, and Susan and I attended a meeting devoted to the process of Chinese adoption. One of the highlights of the program was meeting families who had returned from China in months and years past and their daughters. Susan's and my eyes streamed with tears as we saw the little girls make their way through the audience, smiling and then running back to the arms of their parents. The whole adoption process required only one trip that lasted ten days and we could travel in a group with other adoptive parents.

I noticed that one of the names on a list of previous adoptive families was that of a professor whom I knew from my doctoral training program. I called her on the telephone and she relayed her wonderful experiences with the agency and adopting her children from China. It was after that telephone call that Susan and I knew that we were going to China to adopt our second daughter.

In 2000, adopting a child in China was certainly not for anyone afraid of paperwork. For two months we went through an application process that involved every conceivable background check into our lives. The stability of our employment was verified and we spent many hours notarizing the many forms that had to be filled out. We collected tax returns, bank statements, affidavits of health from our physicians, blood tests, attestations as to our character, fingerprints, and underwent a thorough home study by a social worker—all to insure that the environment and resources that we had to offer were suitable for a new baby. Fortunately, our family provided not only emotional but also financial support since the cost of adoption including the trip to China to meet our child would be more than $20,000.

In October of 2000, we received word from the adoption agency that our packet had been received and forwarded to the authorities in China. There, the documents would be translated into Chinese. We would then have to wait from ten to twelve months to find out whether we would be able to adopt a child.

With Chinese adoptions, parents do not select the child that they are going to adopt. Instead, the Chinese government has an agency that matches children with potential adoptive families. In the literature that I had read, it seemed as if everything from the pictures of the prospective parents, their written narrative about why they wanted to adopt, and the recommendations of the social workers were all considered in matching parents with an appropriate child. Susan and I did not know who would be selected for us, but we reasoned that when you have a biological child, you never know what type of personality will be brought into the world. It wouldn't be that different with adopting from China. What we knew for sure was that no matter what child was selected, we would love her as much as any biological child.

The months passed and the waiting became increasingly difficult. We wondered about when our future daughter had been born and where she lived. We found ourselves anguished at the thought of her being alone, in institutional care, not knowing that across the globe there were loving parents who longed to hold her and to let her know that she was not just one of scores of tiny orphans in an institution, but someone very special and precious.

In the meantime, we joined a discussion group on the Internet for parents from all over the world who had sent their materials (referred to as dossiers) to China. This provided a wonderful forum for parents waiting to travel to China to exchange information and share their concerns as well as their joy when they obtained good news about their child. As people received information about their children, they shared referral pictures or information about their travel plans to China. This inspired others in the group who had been waiting anxiously for information. Occasionally, we would actually hear exciting news from parents who were actually in China at that moment or who had just returned. We marveled in hearing about what it was like for someone to finally meet and to hold their new child.

It was not until 13 months later that we learned the identity of our daughter. It was November of 2001 and Rachel had just celebrated her sixth birthday. Every day for over a year, we had waited to hear word about our new daughter. Finally, the day arrived when we received the exciting telephone call from the adoption agency. We were told that the agency had just received the information about the child that had been selected for us and that the information and pictures of the child would be sent overnight by Federal Express.

Susan and I could barely contain our excitement. I took the day off from work and we waited for the delivery truck to arrive. The next morning we heard a knock on the door and ran to retrieve the precious large envelope. Susan's hands trembled as she opened it and there was a picture of our second daughter. She was being held in front of the camera, and stared at us with big brown and soulful eyes. She was sucking on her left hand and could not have been more than six months of age. She was not smiling and looked shy. Sue turned to a report that read "Children Medical Examination Record," but the entire report was in Chinese. Fortunately, another copy in the folder had been translated into English.

We learned that our daughter Amy was found in front of an orphanage in Anhui province at six weeks of age with nothing more than a blanket and the date of her birth. She was in good health and was described as a very alert and curious child. She was 11 months old. She was described in glowing terms but the description included one line stating that Amy would get "angry if the other babies were fed before she was fed." "I wonder if Amy has a temper," mused Susan, with tears of joy. At that time she did not know the half of it, as we would find out later.

Susan and I held each other and shared our joy in our embrace. We now had three pictures of Amy and an entire medical and social report describing her developmental history. Suddenly, the concept of having a daughter was no longer abstract but was definitely real. Our daughter was in an orphanage in Anquing City, in Anhui Province. Looking at a world map, we found that Anhui was located about half way between Beijing, the capital of China in the northern part of the country, and Guangzhou in the south. We searched the Internet to find as much information as we could about where our daughter lived. Our daughter was half a world away in a largely rural province that was one of the greatest exporters of rice to the rest of China.

Susan and I were very happy and relieved to learn that our daughter's orphanage was widely acknowledged for the excellence of its care for children. In addition to an attentive staff, it had a grandmother's program through which women in the community came in and spent time with the children, holding and rocking them. Susan and I were touched that such attention was paid to providing extra individualized attention to the children.

Several days later we learned that we would soon be traveling to China and shortly had airline tickets for travel to Detroit, Michigan on the seventh of December. There we would join ten other adoptive families and take the 13-hour flight from Detroit to Beijing. The group would spend one day in Beijing and then split apart. Our group would fly to Hefei, the capital city of Anhui province. We would then wait in our hotel as our daughters traveled with their caretakers by bus to meet us.

There was much to do in preparing for our trip and little time in which to do it. Susan and I enlisted the aid of all of our family members, who would take turns staying with Rachel. She was well aware that she was going to have a sister and seemed quite excited about it. We also had hired a very nice lady to help our parents and siblings attend to Rachel's special needs.

Susan's mom, Doris, and my parents, Arline and Jack, would take turns staying over in our house with Rachel. We were thankful that our in-laws got along so well. Our sisters, Fran and Linda, also had volunteered to help out. With the support of our family and some other help, Susan and I felt that Rachel would be well cared for. We met with Rachel's school officials and helped them to understand that Rachel might require a bit more emotional support, since this was the first time that our family had been separated for any length of time since the days in the NICU.

Susan and I "shopped till we dropped" for all of the baby items that we would be taking to China and for all of the clothes, toys and furniture that Amy would need when we returned home. We also had to get some winter clothes. Susan and I were native Floridians who shuddered when the temperature fell into the 40s or 50s. China in the middle of the winter was going to be a different experience. Susan's sister and a close friend arranged a baby shower. Among those who attended was Dr. Shahnaz Duara, Rachel's godmother.

Flying had never been easy for Susan and she was especially nervous since the attack two months before on the World Trade Center. I had been giving a talk at a professional conference on Alzheimer's disease in Nice, France, at that time and had been unable to come home for several days because of flight cancellations. Susan's determination to fly in spite of her anxiety was a testament to just how much she wanted to hold her daughter.

The Loewensteins are noted for over packing for trips, and the biggest trip of our life was no exception. We packed and unpacked our bags several times but finally we got everything to fit. "Sue!" I exclaimed. "We've packed enough so that we could live in China for a year!" She gave me a playful shove. "Shut up if you know what's good for you."

On the day that we were to leave, Susan and I gathered Rachel into our arms and asked her if she knew what day it was. Rachel broke into a big grin. "This is the day that you are going to fly to China to pick up my little sister." She slid her tiny glasses back over her nose and said slowly, "Mommy and Daddy, I'm really going to miss you."

We all hugged so tightly that it seemed as if we would never let go. Grandma Doris took Rachel into the other room and started playing, and my parents helped us pack our car and drove us to the Fort Lauderdale airport. As we made our way there, I looked out the window and wondered what our daughter was doing at that very moment. China was on the other side of the world and it was 13 hours later there than in the United States. At that moment, Amy was probably sleeping, unaware that in a few days her life was going to change dramatically. Her parents were beginning their travels from the other side of the world to bring her home.

Chapter Ten

VOYAGE TO CHINA

I HAD READ THAT RIDING in economy class for 13 hours could be tough. At six feet tall, I had to agree. I walked around the plane every couple of hours to keep the blood circulating. It was exciting to talk to other prospective parents from all over the country who were embarking on the same exciting odyssey. All of us were flying to a faraway land, to visit a people and a culture very different from our own. Over the last month Susan and I had read books trying to learn some simple Chinese phrases. A colleague had also taught me how to successfully use chopsticks, no small feat for me.

During the flight, Susan and I periodically looked at pictures of Amy and were shown pictures of the other waiting children by proud adoptive parents. As the plane took us across the ocean and numerous time zones, our excitement and anticipation increased. When we finally landed, it was evening in Beijing. We waited with as much patience as we could muster as we were processed through customs and then taken to a hotel. The next day we would tour the city. Having been born in Florida, Susan and I found it was difficult to get used to the snow and the winter temperatures that were in the 20s and low 30s. When we gathered in the lobby for the tour, it certainly wasn't hard to identify the Floridians—you only had to listen for the sound of chattering teeth.

In the morning, we visited the Forbidden City in the middle of Beijing. Snow lay on the ground as far as we could see. Uniformed soldiers stood on street corners and in front of many monuments and entrances to buildings. There are almost 10,000 buildings within the Forbidden City, so it is easy to become lost. We followed our tour guide and gazed at the wondrous architecture beyond the Meridian Gate at the southern entrance to the Forbidden City. Since Chinese emperors had believed that they were sons of the universe, they believed that they should live in the meridian, the true center of the universe. Susan and I marveled at the buildings, architecture and the artwork. As we approached Tiananmen, we came to the main gate of the Outer Court which was guarded by two impressive bronze statues of lions. The palace was magnificent and unlike anything we had ever seen.

Later, we were taken by bus to the Great Wall of China. From the north to northwest of Beijing, this serrated wall goes from east to west across the mountains. Construction of the Great Wall began in the seventh century B.C. and it was designed to be used for defense against invaders. The Great Wall is so large that it is the only man-made structure that can be seen from the moon. The opportunity to climb the steps of the Great Wall of China was quite exciting. A number of the people in our tour climbed for about 20 minutes, a sufficient distance to reach the souvenir store to purchase shirts and other mementos. I was determined that if I was privileged enough to have the opportunity to climb the Great Wall of China then that was what I was going to do. The cold thin air made it difficult for me to catch my breath as I ascended higher and higher. As I made my way to the upper levels of the wall, young Chinese university students in their teens and twenties asked if I would take pictures of them. They did not speak English, but somehow through our smiles and gestures we were able to communicate. When I finally reached the top of the wall I looked down on the cars and buses far below. They were just dots. The beautiful scene was breathtaking and I went to several different locations to take pictures.

Lost in my appreciation of the beautiful surroundings, I took the wrong path on the way down from the Wall. I wandered from the more widely-used public path to one that was older. It had been used thousands of years before to descend from the mountain. Unfortunately, by the time I reached the ground, there was no sign of our bus and I couldn't find anyone who spoke English. By the time I found our bus it had been a 20-minute walk.

Everyone else was seated and ready to go. Although I had returned ten minutes earlier than our scheduled departure time, everyone else in our party had been ready to leave for 20 minutes. I thought Susan would kill me, but, luckily for me, there were witnesses present.

That night in the hotel I found it painful to breathe. "I think with the cold thin air I may have burst a few air sacs in my lungs," I told Susan. She wasn't sympathetic.

"Listen, David, we've gone all the way around the world to adopt our daughter and you climb so high under winter conditions that you could have killed yourself! I haven't traveled all this way for Rachel and Amy to be without a father." I hung my head and stopped complaining.

The next day was the ninth of December, 2001, and our adoption group divided in two. About half of the prospective parents would fly to Guandong Province, while five prospective families would fly to Anhui Province. Several hours later, Susan and I were on a plane with the four other adoptive families on our way to Hefei, the capital of Anhui Province. The plane ride south took a little more than two hours. When we touched down we were taken to a beautiful hotel in the center of the city.

The view of Hefei from our hotel was magnificent. It was striking how few cars there were on the streets compared to the number of persons walking or on bicycles. The streets were bustling and vibrant. Our observations of the city were interrupted by a knock on the hotel room door. Someone had come to tell us that there would be a gathering of all the adoptive parents in our group that evening.

At the meeting, we were introduced to our adoption guide who also served as our translator. She was accompanied by a physician who would be available if needed for any of the babies. Since we would not visit the orphanage in Anqing, we were told the details of how our children would be brought to us in the hotel. We reviewed the procedures and paperwork that had to be filed with local authorities after our child arrived. Nobody in our group was able to contain their excitement as we were told that we would meet our

children the next day. We would then begin
local adoption proceedings. Later that night
we talked by telephone to Rachel and her
grandparents, sharing the exciting news. Our
older daughter greatly missed us but looked
forward to our calls in the evenings. Being
with grandparents and other family members
allowed Rachel to continue with school and
her daily routine without any difficulty.

At nine the next morning we gathered in
a large conference room with several Chinese
officials. A few minutes later we were informed
that the bus had been delayed, but that the
children and the orphanage attendants would
arrive in 40 minutes. Finally, just as it seemed
that we could wait no longer, the first baby
came through the double doors carried by a
young woman who worked at the orphanage.
Her parents cried with joy and rushed to their
new daughter. Then two babies were carried
through the door by attendants. The baby
on the left was unmistakably Amy. Susan
and I ran to her and hugged her for the longest time. Amy's diaper was wet and Susan
happily performed her first responsibility as

a new mother. Amy had the most beautiful face with big brown eyes and chubby cheeks. At just under a year of age, she had a full head of straight dark hair. Susan and I took turns holding Amy as the adoption papers were processed. Later, we were permitted to take Amy to our room to spend time getting to know each another.

Since we had read that adopted babies could be reluctant to immediately bond with new parents, we were amazed at how easily Amy took to both Susan and me. She was quite comfortable with being held and actually fell asleep while lying on my chest. She refused to take formula unless it was sweetened with sugar—apparently, milk in the orphanage had been sweetened with cane sugar. We also noted that Amy didn't get around very well when crawling. Fortunately, we had been told that babies from Chinese orphanages sometimes initially seemed developmentally delayed but that they caught up quickly after adoption.

For the next several days in Hefei while papers were being processed, our group went on outings with our daughters so that we could experience Chinese culture. We visited an elementary school and were serenaded by children in kindergarten. We toured museums, historic landmarks and shopping areas. We had lunch and dinner in different types of Chinese restaurants to experience different dishes. In one restaurant I tried camel hump which was tough and fatty. It definitely did not taste like chicken. I stayed away from some of the other exotic delicacies including snake.

In the evenings, we would spend time alone with Amy and e-mail pictures to the family back home. On quiet days while Susan and Amy were napping, I wandered the streets, going into different neighborhoods to get a better sense of both the people and culture. I was struck by the large number of child and elderly beggars. When I gave them money, more children and adults would pour into the streets asking me for money. I quickly ran out of cash but was still poked and prodded by these unfortunate people who were pleading for anything I could spare. As the crowd grew larger around me, I ducked into a three-story department store that was guarded by a soldier. He spoke sternly to them in Chinese and they began to disperse. I stayed in the department store for more than 45 minutes to make sure that I wouldn't be followed on the way back to the hotel.

It was interesting how protective the Chinese people were of children. If anyone felt that a child was not bundled up correctly he or she would race over to cover that child's skin.

As we went to different parts of Hefei, we were stopped many times by people who admired Amy's beauty. Anquing City bordered the Yangtze River and our Chinese friends told us that the area was home to some of the most tall and beautiful women in China. It was impossible, however, to know whether Amy had actually been born in Anquing City, since abandoned children were sometimes found hundreds of miles from where they had actually been born.

On Amy's first birthday, I took a cab to a book and card store to purchase a candle for a celebration. The taxi driver helpfully accompanied me inside to help translate. I was very grateful and left a tip equivalent to at least a week's pay for the average person in China. Susan and I celebrated her birthday together in the hotel buffet and dining room. We placed the candle in a small cupcake and sang as tears rolled down our faces. Amy was much less impressed with our singing than the taste of the cupcake.

Our group next flew from Anhui Province south to Guangzhou to rejoin the rest of our group. It was a joyful reunion for the families. We visited with each other and admired the treasures that we had just adopted. Adoptive parents from all over China are required to go to the American Embassy at Guangzhou to prepare the papers that allow them to re-enter the United States. At that time our country had just passed a law granting immediate citizenship to all adopted Chinese children of United States citizens when they came to the U.S. When we landed in Detroit, Michigan, and passed through customs, our daughter Amy officially became a U.S. citizen.

It was finally homecoming day. When we approached the door of our house we were excited about being home and about the chance to introduce Amy Michelle Loewenstein to the family. We were also extremely anxious to see Rachel whom we had missed desperately.

As the door opened, Rachel flew out and held on to Susan and me as though her life depended on it. She was crying.

"Please don't ever go away again, Mommy and Daddy. I missed you so much!" We held Rachel and told her that we would never leave her again. Now more calm, Rachel then proceeded to go into the living room to size up her new sister.

Chapter Eleven

ACCEPTANCE
AND ITS GRACE

N O ONE WAS EVER BORN into this world having learned prejudice or hate. These are, unfortunately, taught by persons who have not learned very much in their own lives. Those who truly accept their common humanity do not exclude people because they have a different amount of melanin in their skins, belong to a different cultural background or have different religious practices. Similarly, a physical or a mental disability does not make a person any less real or their needs any less legitimate. These human beings long to experience success and a sense of accomplishment, just as we all do. When they are physically hurt, these individuals bleed like the rest of us. At those times when they are isolated or rejected, these people feel the same pain and experience the same despair as does any other person on this planet.

The experience of Rachel's birth and subsequent disabilities made me grateful for the openness and acceptance of my own parents and the privilege of working with special needs children in my youth. It was actually my experience with a special needs child that first motivated me to pursue a career in a helping profession. I was in the seventh grade and had volunteered to work in the special education department with adolescents who had a variety of special needs. One boy was extremely bright, but his cerebral palsy gave him the inability to control his body or his speech. A number of other children suffered from mental retardation. The person who was assigned to me must have been 16 or 17 years of age. Joseph had been a normal child when as a toddler he was struck by a car. He was now confined to a wheelchair with braces on his legs that enabled him to take a few steps with assistance. He was mentally retarded and his speech was slurred. When he talked, Joseph sounded as if he were three or four years of age. If Joseph had not been disabled, he could well have been a defensive lineman on a high school football team. He was very big and extremely strong. My assignment was to help Joseph as he drew, put puzzles together, and help wheel him to the bathroom. Each afternoon, when I was able, I worked with him and began to learn that beneath the physical disability and mental retardation was a magnificent human being. Joseph had a heart of gold and would greet every child and teacher whom he met with a smile. Just being with Joseph and his unbridled optimism was a gift. His disposition was always cheery and his smile would light up a room. I also learned that he was extremely sensitive. He would become quite upset when others teased or made fun of him. Joseph felt sad on days that I could not come and work with him. He loved to smile and his laugh was infectious. Recently, I came across an old poem that I had written when I was perhaps 13 years of age and working with Joseph. It brought back memories...

Gazing into eyes of sensitivity and warmth, one cannot help but to feel pity for him.

Determination gripping his face, he tries to fit a children's puzzle in the right space.

Seconds turn into minutes as that look of determination is replaced by a look of frustration as he slides the puzzle pieces aimlessly across the board.

You feel the urge to help him solve this mystery which holds him spellbound, but you know that he must feel the thrill of accomplishment.

He tries to control his hands as he lays them on your shoulder.

You try to understand him but it is very hard.

However, there is one thing that you can understand, the smile and feeling of warmth because you know that you and he are friends…

Most importantly is the feeling inside when you come to know that one human being helping another is what life is all about.

My thoughts had turned to Joseph when Rachel, then aged two years, put her hand on my shoulder and cooed, repeating the sound "dada." Susan and I had consulted a number of speech therapists who were uncertain whether Rachel would be able to talk normally. I looked into Rachel's dancing but soulful brown eyes and reveled in her laughter. Like Joseph, Rachel had a wonderful disposition and an infectious smile. Despite living her early life in an incubator, she loved to be held and cuddled. There was something about her that was so innocent, pure and lovable—traits that she possesses to this day.

Learning to accept the challenges and limitations of special needs children is a task that the children and family members constantly face. However, in the end, the grace of acceptance can be quite enlightening and can serve to foster our personal and spiritual growth as human beings. To finally accept the limitations of a child who was supposed to be imbued with endless possibilities is to learn to also accept the inherent limitations within ourselves and others around us. To understand that we all struggle with our limitations and fallibility is to finally embrace our true humanity. In professional baseball, an accomplished player may have a batting average of 0.300. However, that means that he only successfully reaches base three times in ten at bat. Being less than perfect is certainly sufficient in the major leagues. Hundreds of scientists may work on cures for the amelioration of certain diseases and encounter many blind alleys. In reality, there are only a few scientists who actually make unique and ground-breaking discoveries. That does not diminish the efforts of others in trying to further the human good or the value of them laying down the necessary bricks to build the foundation upon which discoveries can be made. Despite medical science's efforts at trying to prolong and to preserve life, all of us will eventually wither and die. Our bodies are not perfect, nor are our lives.

The lives of physically and mentally challenged children are no less valuable than the lives of others who have faced lesser challenges. In fact, the inspiration that we can derive from their struggles and victories of the body as well as the spirit can inspire us to look beyond the superficial, material and trivial things in this world to which we often ascribe so much importance.

The parents of special needs children frequently need to be reminded to not be overly critical of themselves when they occasionally become impatient or intolerant of their children. What is important is to have a reasonable batting average, which can be less than 100%. I remember feeling guilty when I became impatient with Rachel or when I was less than totally understanding. Something that she wrote about me in the 4th grade helps remind me to this day that, despite my flaws, my batting average was adequate:

My Dad

by Rachel Loewenstein

My Dad is a super Dad. He is very special to me. He is the best Dad in the whole world. Dad always makes me very happy. To begin with, he provides us with clothes and a house for us to live. He gives our family all the things we need and most of the things we want.

My Dad spends a lot of time with me. He talks to me about doing good and being the best I can be. He helps me do my homework. He works with me on my computer. He teaches me math. He reads to me and I read to him. He is helping me plan my future.

In addition, he always makes me happy by telling me jokes and he calls me a nickname "Rach" and he makes funny faces and says funny things that make me laugh. We watch Letter Factory videos and cartoons together. When I am very good he takes me to Toys 'R' Us to buy me toys.

In conclusion, these are just a few of reasons why my Dad is someone very special to me and I love him and he loves me.

To fully accept a person in spite of physical or mental limitations is to truly embrace our humanity. I have come to believe that trying to mainstream special needs children in both public and private schools benefits not only the children, but greatly benefits their class-mates as well. Children are by nature some of the most accepting creatures in the universe until they are taught to fear those who are different from them or, even worse, learn to hate. By discovering that a special needs child is part of their world and deserving of friend-ship and respect, other children learn a most valuable lesson, one that certainly cannot be learned from textbooks alone.

Human beings have historically been fearful of those who are different from them-selves. We have also learned to fear things in ourselves such as anger, imperfection and our physical, cognitive and emotional limitations that keep us from realizing the idealized images we have of ourselves. However, the acceptance of our limitations and failings can also lead us to a greater appreciation of other gifts that are often taken for granted. Living with a special needs child has taught me to accept the fact that I cannot always be right, nor can I always be wise or patient. Winston

Churchill once proclaimed, "I am always willing to learn, however, I do not always like to be taught."

Being the father of a child with cognitive and physical limitations has taught me that outer appearances tell us little of what is important. It is far easier to judge and to skim the surface of people and important issues than to explore the truth that lies underneath. Particularly troubling is the lack of acceptance of different points of view. It is far easier to be close-minded and judgmental in our society, rather than sitting down and honestly airing our differences and finding common ground on which we can work. Politics seems to be more about big money, special interests and creating slogans that polarize rather than bringing people together. There seems to be less emphasis on obtaining truth than on "spinning" the perceptions of the average person in the fast-paced world in which we live.

Rachel's birth and her residual disabilities made me realize what was truly important to me, and I realized that my family was even more important than the work I so loved. I learned to place an even greater value on integrity and compassion. Rather than just listening to people, I tried to truly hear not only with my ears and brain but with my heart. My daughter's physical challenges were also constant reminders to me about my own physical limitations. I was accustomed to working 16 hour days and focusing my entire life on my research productivity. Now, I realized that moments that I did not spend with Rachel and my family were moments that would be lost forever. If I did not take care of my physical and emotional health, I might risk a greater chance of dying early and leaving Rachel, Susan and Amy in a very precarious position. My own father had a stroke at 52 years of age that ended his career as a scientist and a very successful acoustical engineer. He was far smarter than I and was an extremely conscientious and hard worker. Fortunately, he had carefully planned his financial future and had successfully launched his children. Mom was an accomplished child psychologist who had a leadership position in the public school system and continued to work. What would happen to Susan, Rachel and Amy were I to become ill or disabled? This caused me to rethink some of my priorities—something that I probably would not have considered if Rachel's situation had not knocked me off "automatic pilot."

The acceptance of the limitations of a special needs child provides us with the opportunity to reflect upon the many gifts that we may sometimes fail to appreciate. It is far too easy to take things for granted, such as our ability to see, hear, speak, work, remember and reason. When these things are taken away, we finally come to realize the value of the gifts that have been bestowed upon us. It is also easy to feel overly sorry for oneself if one does not realize that misfortunes, particularly for a person in the United States, are so much smaller than those experienced by many people in other parts of the world. Despite our sometimes irrational insistence, life is not always fair. The universe does not always unfold to meet our particular needs.

To accept the physical and the cognitive challenges of our children, to love them unconditionally, and to relinquish the illusion of living vicariously through their accomplishments is often the greatest challenge that a parent must learn to accept. If we can realize that a child with physical and mental disabilities is just as uniquely human and valuable as any other child, we can also come to a new understanding: regardless of special need, pigment of skin or cultural or religious background, these children and the adults they become deserve our love and respect.

As I write these pages, my thoughts turn to the sense of unity and solidarity of all of the parents who had children in the NICU. They came from every ethnic, cultural and language background imaginable. Some were quite socioeconomically well off while others were quite poor. However, we were all united in the love for our children and our solidarity in their struggle for survival. Perhaps there is a lesson there for all of us. When we are united by our common humanity, solving the problems that confront all of us becomes more important than our differences. The politicians and policy makers of this country could learn much from the tiniest babies and their families.

Chapter Twelve

TODAY AND TOMORROW

It HAS BEEN NEARLY 12 YEARS since Rachel's birth at 510 grams, or about 18 ounces. Since then, considerable progress has been made in saving the tiniest babies, premature infants weighing 1,000 grams or less. In addition, improvements in early treatment have reduced the chances of significant disability. Early intervention is critical since follow-up studies on premature infants indicate that as a group, they are at greater risk for physical disability as well as different types of cognitive and learning deficits. Thanks to the efforts and dedication of countless clinicians and research investigators, the outlook for these tiny warriors has substantially improved. In addition to treatments for infants that are born prematurely, there have also been increased efforts at developing effective interventions to reduce the risk of prematurity itself.

Unfortunately, despite all of our technological advances, it has been impossible to create an environment for the premature infant that even approaches those nurturing and protective conditions within the womb. Infants born with less than 20 weeks gestation still have little realistic chance of survival. Premature babies are still at much greater risk for cerebral palsy, chronic respiratory problems, cardiac abnormalities, vision and hearing loss, and failure to thrive (from both a physical and a cognitive perspective) relative to their full-term counterparts. This is especially true of those micro-premies born at 1,000 grams or less.

I have heard some people who question the social and economic costs associated with saving our tiniest babies. They put forth the argument that many sick children were never meant by nature to survive. If one were to strictly adhere to this line of reasoning then society's efforts to help people who have sustained neurological conditions such as stroke or closed head injury could be equally assailed. Millions of persons with chronic medical conditions such as diabetes, renal disease or congestive heart failure have been kept alive and have been able to add years to their lives and quality to their years. Why should our precious children, if there is a chance of viability, not have a similar opportunity?

In the United States, we spend billions of dollars for cosmetic surgery and pills to enhance our sexual performance and rarely consider that far more money is spent in our desire to look and feel good than to eradicate prematurity or develop more effective treatments for too many of our children born early or full-term with life threatening illnesses. I only have to look in Rachel's eyes to know the value of the work that Shahnaz and other neonatology professionals provide to our communities.

Rachel will be entering the sixth grade and, with the help of a wonderful aide, has been able to keep up with a normal class curriculum. My oldest daughter wears thick glasses because of severe myopia and she has loss of peripheral vision because of the scarring that occurred with her retinopathy. She wears bilateral hearing aids because of auditory loss discovered when she was six years of age, likely caused by some of the medications that were administered to keep her alive. Rachel continues to have difficulties chewing solid foods and Pediasure, a nutritional supplement, has been a mainstay of her diet. Rachel's visual deficits, coupled with mild cerebral palsy and missing digits and thumb on her right hand, make it difficult for her to button and zip clothing. However, she refuses to be defined by these limitations. Her sweet disposition and engaging smile has endeared her to her classmates, teachers, and to everyone who meets her. She is very affectionate and has a wonderful sense of humor. The teachers and staff at Rachel's school have been outstanding. As wonderful as the school experience has been for Rachel, the children around her have also benefited. By interacting with Rachel since she was in kindergarten, they have learned a precious lesson that physical disability and unevenness in cognitive strengths and weaknesses does not change the essence of one's humanity. Rachel exhibits a positive attitude in the face of the challenges that confront her. In the words of her grandfather, "Rachel is like a bumblebee. A bumblebee aerodynamically should not be able to fly but it does." Rachel is the proverbial bumblebee. She should not be able to do many of the things that she does. However she doesn't know that she is supposed to be unable to do them. As Shahnaz Duara is fond of saying, "Rachel writes her own book."

Life has not been without its challenges or uncertainties. In the first several years after she came home, Rachel had some seizure activity. Two years ago, after a seizure, an MRI of her brain revealed what appeared to a number of physicians to be a neoplasm, a small astrocytoma near the brain stem. However, after several follow-up scans the lesion has not progressed and actually has looked smaller. As a result, the experts have the opinion that this might be scarring left over from an inflammatory process. The MRI scan intervals have now been pushed back to once per year, and every time we receive encouraging results we breathe somewhat easier.

Rachel has had a number of wonderful therapists at the Dan Marino Center in Weston, Florida, where she has worked on her chewing, articulation, and dressing skills. These and other areas require continual attention. Susan and I have concerns about the future. Our most important goals as parents are to give Rachel the tools and every advantage so that she can enjoy a high quality of life with maximum autonomy and independence.

Amy recently turned six years old and she is a very happy, bubbly and playful child. When she first came home, she was plagued with numerous ear infections, eventually necessitating the surgical implantation of ear tubes. Her ENT physician tells us it is fortunate that Amy was treated since it is likely that she would have become deaf if this issue had not been addressed. While there is occasionally sibling rivalry, Amy adores her sister Rachel and the feeling is definitely mutual.

Whereas her older sister likes computers and anything electronic, Amy is partial to dolls and likes to dress up like a princess. Both girls are beautiful like their mother. Amy is very loving but quite an independent spirit. I remember picking her up from preschool at four years of age and asking her about her day. She smiled, crossed her arms and then replied, "Daddy, I don't want to talk about it." More recently, when I was picking her up from kindergarten Amy got into the car and turned to me and excitedly exclaimed, "Daddy, I have found that there is a voice in my head so that I can think things that other people can't hear." She continued, "Do you want to know what the voice inside of my head says when you tell me something?" "What is that?" I asked quizzically. Amy shrugged her shoulders and grinned, ""Blah, blah, blah. Whatever!" I could barely contain my laughter. If my daughter was this irreverent at five years of age, I could only imagine what adolescence would bring.

Susan and I are approaching our 15th wedding anniversary. Although it doesn't seem possible, I grow to love and to appreciate her more every day. The philosopher Nietzsche once wrote that those things which do not destroy you make you stronger. We never wanted to confront some of the horrible experiences that we have faced, but we both believe that the experience has strengthened us and has taught us lessons that we might have never appreciated. Kahlil Gibran, the philosopher and poet, wrote in his book *The Prophet* that our pain may be likened to clay. The clay that the potter digs into the deepest often forms the vessel that can ultimately hold the most wine. I don't know if Susan's and my experiences have provided us with the potential for more happiness, but I do know that we both have a greater appreciation for all of the blessings that have been bestowed upon us. The four ingredients that keep our relationship strong and vibrant are love, respect, trust and communication. We believe that these are the foundations from which everything in our marriage flows. Perhaps someday we will write about it. Susan and I have also been fortunate to have the services of United Cerebral

Palsy (UCP), which provides us with respite services so that we can have some alone time, a movie, dinner out or an evening with friends. Relationships are like gardens that need to be tended. We are grateful that respite programs such as those provided by UCP are available to parents in the area in which we live.

I believe that the circumstances surrounding Rachel's birth and our journey to China to bring Amy home have resulted in a special relationship with both of my daughters. Recently, Rachel had a writing assignment in school. She brought it home and Susan left it on my pillow. It had been a hard day at work and I was incredibly touched when I read my daughter's prose:

10/23/06   Ms. T Writing

I Am Thankful For My Dad

By Rachel Loewenstein

My Dad's name is David Loewenstein. He is my favorite person in the world. He is smart and he always teaches things, he does things with me. We have lots of fun together and I am proud and thankful to have him as my dad. Dad is very smart, he is a doctor in Miami. He takes care of people and helps them to get better. He takes care of me and my little sister Amy. Even when I'm not feeling good, he makes me smile, laugh, and feel better.

My dad works with me on the computer and teaches me how to press Enter. He helps me to set up e-mail, change fonts, and listen to music all on the computer. He helps me with my homework, reads with me. We go to fun places and do fun things together like swimming, watch cartoons, walking and playing games. He takes me to Disney World, Busch Gardens, musical shows and to the zoo. When I'm very good my dad buys me toys and presents.

These are all the things that make my dad, my favorite person in the world. I love him because he is smart and because of all the things he does for me. I am lucky and very thankful to have him be my dad.

To know that my love and nurturance has had a positive impact on Rachel is far more precious than gold. Parents can only hope to provide good launching pads so that children can become the unique individuals that they have the potential to be. No one knows what the future holds for any of us, but Susan and I can be take comfort in the knowledge that Rachel feels secure and very much loved.

In fairy tales, the story ends with "happily ever after." Unfortunately, our family does not know exactly how all of life's challenges will play out. Rachel and Amy will both have to face issues regarding the unique circumstances of their arrival into the world. Rachel will have to continually deal with issues regarding her physical limitations. As her coursework becomes more difficult and abstract, in the years ahead she may yet face further cognitive and academic challenges. Amy may come to question her heritage and her roots in China. Both of my children face potential issues because they may perceive themselves to be somewhat different from others. Nonetheless, Susan and I hope that they will ultimately realize that, in addition to our common humanity, it is our diversity and our differences that make us unique and special. Like most parents, we are worried about ballooning federal deficits, dependence on foreign oil and damage to the environment that may mortgage and compromise their futures. The culture in which we live is all too obsessed with superficial appearance, style over substance, and slogans rather than well-thought-out solutions. Often, there is such an emphasis placed upon winning and competition that we forget that the uniquely human attribute of advanced language and reasoning skills can also be employed to foster cooperation among people and work that insures the common good.

I have been asked about the single most important lesson that I have learned based on Rachel's heroic struggles. Upon reflection, I would have to say that Rachel's journey has taught me that we often never appreciate a blessing until it is lost. Life is a precious gift and no one in the world is guaranteed anything but the present moment. Every human being has been allotted only a finite number of moments that become the foundations of our lives. We never truly know what the future might bring, or how many moments we will be blessed to share with those whom we love. The present moment is a precious gift that each of us is granted to express our love and appreciation to others, live our values and ideals, and make amends or extend forgiveness. We have today. Nobody can guarantee that we will ever get another chance tomorrow.

Rachel has inspired me to embrace the present moment and live, laugh, and love. Too much of our lives are spent stuck in the past or overly preoccupied with anxiety about the future. I wish all of the readers touched by Rachel's journey the greatest gift of all: many precious moments filled with love, wonder and gratitude.